Explaining Endometriosis

Explaining Endometriosis

Second edition

LORRAINE HENDERSON AND ROS WOOD

ALLEN & UNWIN

First published in 1991
This edition published in 2000 by
Allen & Unwin
9 Atchison Street
St Leonards NSW 2065
Australia
Phone: (61 2) 8425 0100
Fax: (61 2) 9906 2218
Email: frontdesk@allen-unwin.com.au
Web: http://www.allen-unwin.com.au

National Library of Australia
Cataloguing-in-Publication entry:

Henderson, Lorraine, 1952–.
 Explaining endometriosis.

 2nd ed.
 Bibliography.
 Includes Index.
 ISBN 1 86508 133 7.

 1. Endometriosis—Diagnosis. 2. Endometriosis—Treatment.
 I. Wood, Ros, 1955–. II. Title.

618.142

Set in 11.5/14 pt Garamond by DOCUPRO, Sydney
Printed and bound by Kin Keong Printing Co. Pte Ltd, Singapore

10 9 8 7 6 5 4 3 2 1

Contents

Preface

Endometriosis can be a difficult condition to live with, but access to accurate and up-to-date information will allow you to cope better. Although more information on endometriosis is now available than when we wrote the first edition of the book, it is still difficult for women to obtain all the information they want. We have rewritten the book to provide you with the latest information.

The content of this book has been developed on the basis of the information we would have liked when we were first diagnosed with the condition and the questions we have been asked by thousands of women during our years with the Endometriosis Association (Victoria). We hope the information will give you the knowledge you need to understand your condition and its implications, and to make well-informed decisions about its management.

The first chapter provides a brief overview of the anatomy and function of the female reproductive system to familiarise you with the terms and concepts that will be used in later chapters. This overview is followed by a number of chapters that look at endometriosis, its diagnosis and treatments. Specialist chapters discuss feelings and emotions, taking control, teenagers and endometriosis, infertility and pregnancy. The last chapter has been written for partners, families and friends to help them support you.

We acknowledge the invaluable advice and support of the Endometriosis Association (Victoria) staff, Lyn Boag, Glenda Cagliarini, Rae Cagliarini, Stella Coniglio, Anne Grendon, Dr Martin Healey, Rebecca Heitbaum, Narelle Henderson,

Dr Dan Kaplan, Dr Mac Talbot, Shelley Wickham, Verle Wood and Tristen Woods. We would like to thank our respective families for their understanding, help and support.

Lorraine Henderson
Ros Wood
2000

1
Female reproductive system

The purpose of this chapter is to provide basic information about the female reproductive system and the
menstrual cycle to help you to better understand the
material in subsequent chapters.

Female reproductive organs

The female reproductive organs consist of the uterus, fallopian tubes, ovaries, cervix, vagina, vulva, clitoris and
labia.

Uterus (womb)

The uterus is a hollow muscular organ about the size
and shape of a flattened pear. It lies between the bladder
and the lower end of the bowel. It measures approximately 7.5 centimetres in length and weighs about
40 grams.

The upper part of the uterus can move forwards and
backwards within the pelvis. Usually it is tilted forwards
so that it lies against the back of the bladder. In this
position it is said to be anteverted. Sometimes the uterus
is tilted backwards, towards the rectum. When it lies in
this position it is said to be retroverted.

The uterus is made up of three layers. The outer layer
is known as the peritoneum. The middle layer consists
of a thick layer of muscle known as the myometrium. The
inner layer that forms the lining of the uterus is known

as the endometrium. When the endometrium is found outside the uterus it is known as endometriosis.

The main function of the uterus is to protect and nourish the growing foetus during pregnancy.

Fallopian tubes

The fallopian tubes are two fine tubes about 10 centimetres in length. They extend from the upper end of each side of the uterus.

The finger-like ends of the fallopian tubes, known as the fimbriae, lie close to and curve around the ovaries. When ovulation occurs one of the fimbria draws the egg into the fallopian tube, which then propels it to the uterus.

Ovaries

The two ovaries lie close to the ends of the fallopian tubes. They are about the size and shape of a brazil nut, being 2.5–3.5 centimetres long and about 1.2 centimetres thick.

The ovaries contain thousands of tiny sacs called ovarian follicles. Each follicle contains an egg, which is known as the ovum. Once a month under the influence of the menstrual hormones one of these follicles grows and releases its ovum.

Cervix

The cervix is the lowest part of the uterus and is about the size and shape of a small plum. It contains a small canal that connects the uterus and the vagina.

Vagina

The vagina is a thin, elastic-like tube approximately 7.5 centimetres in length that extends from the vulva to the cervix.

Vulva

The vulva is made up of the clitoris, the external opening of the vagina, and the labia.

Clitoris

The clitoris is a small organ made up of erectile tissue that is found at the front end of the vulva.

Labia

The labia are the two folds of skin that surround the entrance to the vagina.

Related structures

There are several other structures and spaces associated with the development and growth of endometriosis.

Pelvic cavity

The pelvic cavity is the space within the pelvic bone that contains the reproductive organs, the bladder and the lower part of the bowel.

Peritoneum

The peritoneum is a thin layer of clingfilm-like tissue that covers the organs within the pelvic cavity. It is a very common site of endometriosis.

Peritoneal fluid

The peritoneal fluid is the lubricating fluid secreted by the peritoneum.

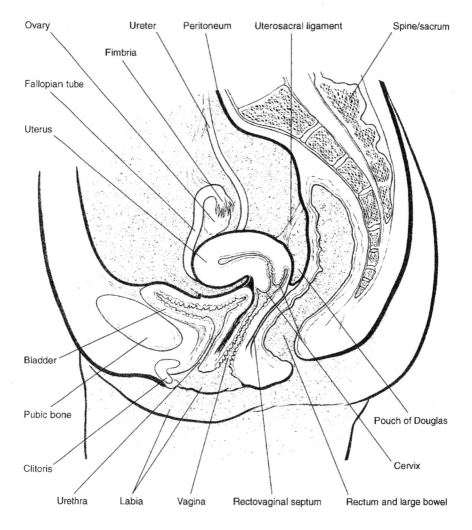

Ovary Ureter Peritoneum Uterosacral ligament Spine/sacrum

Fimbria

Fallopian tube

Uterus

Bladder

Pubic bone

Pouch of Douglas

Clitoris

Cervix

Urethra Labia Vagina Rectovaginal septum Rectum and large bowel

The female reproductive system: side view

Pouch of Douglas

The Pouch of Douglas is the space that lies between the back of the uterus and upper vagina and the front of the lower bowel. It is a common site of endometriosis.

Ligaments

Ligaments are bands of tissue that hold parts of the body in place. The uterus is held in place by four pairs of ligaments: the uterosacral ligaments, the round ligaments, the broad ligaments and the transverse cervical ligaments. The pair most commonly affected by endometriosis are the uterosacral ligaments, which extend from the lower part of the uterus and pass either side of the lower bowel to the inside of the tailbone. The rectovaginal septum is a ligament that lies between the vagina and the rectum below the Pouch of Douglas. It is an occasional site of endometriosis.

Ureters

The ureters are very fine tubes that drain urine from the kidneys into the bladder. Sometimes endometrial implants or nodules lie over the lower part of a ureter.

Pituitary gland

The pituitary gland is a small gland about the size of a pea that lies just below the brain. It releases a variety of hormones that control many of the body's functions, including the menstrual cycle.

Hormones of the menstrual cycle

Hormones are chemicals released by a number of specialised glands in the body, including the pituitary gland. The menstrual cycle is controlled by several hormones, the most important of which are follicle stimulating hormone, luteinising hormone, oestrogen and progesterone.

Follicle stimulating hormone

Follicle stimulating hormone, which is produced by the pituitary gland, stimulates the ovarian follicles to grow and develop.

Luteinising hormone

Luteinising hormone, which is produced by the pituitary gland, initiates ovulation and stimulates the corpus luteum (see page 7) to produce progesterone.

Oestrogen

Oestrogen, which is produced by the ovaries, stimulates the growth of the endometrium.

Progesterone

Progesterone, which is produced by the corpus luteum (see page 7), prepares the endometrium for implantation of the fertilised ovum.

Phases of the menstrual cycle

The menstrual cycle involves a series of hormonal changes that occur at fairly regular intervals. The average menstrual cycle is about 28 days, although this varies considerably between women.

The menstrual cycle involves cyclical changes in both the ovary and the endometrium. The ovarian cycle has two phases: the follicular phase and the luteal phase. The endometrial cycle has three phases: the proliferative phase, the secretory phase, and the menstrual phase.

Follicular phase of ovary

The follicular phase of the ovary begins on the first day of menstruation (the period) and ends on the day of ovulation. During the follicular phase the pituitary gland releases follicle stimulating hormone which stimulates the growth and development of several ovarian follicles in the ovary. These follicles enlarge, mature, and slowly move towards the surface of the ovary. However, only one follicle will reach full maturity.

As the dominant follicle matures it secretes increasing amounts of oestrogen. The oestrogen levels reach a peak after about 14 days. This stimulates the pituitary gland to release a burst of luteinising hormone. The burst of luteinising hormone causes the mature ovarian follicle to rupture and release its ovum through the surface of the ovary. This process is known as ovulation.

Luteal phase of ovary

The luteal phase of the ovary extends from ovulation to the first day of menstruation. Immediately after ovulation the remains of the ruptured ovarian follicle are transformed into a structure known as the corpus luteum. The corpus luteum then begins to secrete progesterone and a small amount of oestrogen.

If fertilisation of the ovum does not occur the corpus luteum degenerates and the levels of progesterone and oestrogen decrease.

Proliferative phase of endometrium

The proliferative phase of the endometrium occurs during the follicular phase of the ovary. The oestrogen secreted by the dominant ovarian follicle stimulates the proliferation (growth and development) of the endometrium so that it is ready to implant a fertilised ovum.

Secretory phase of endometrium

The secretory phase of the endometrium occurs at the same time as the luteal phase of the ovary. The progesterone produced by the corpus luteum stimulates the endometrium to proliferate even more. It also stimulates the cells in the endometrium to secrete substances that will nourish the fertilised ovum if pregnancy occurs.

Menstrual phase of endometrium

The menstrual phase occurs during the late luteal and early follicular phases of the ovary. If the ovum is not fertilised the secretion of progesterone and oestrogen by the corpus luteum decreases. This causes the endometrium to break down and bleed. This bleeding is known as a menstrual period. The menstrual flow consists of blood, endometrial cells, secretions and the unfertilised ovum.

2
What is endometriosis?

Endometriosis is a condition in which endometrium (that is, the lining of the uterus) is found in locations outside the uterus. This chapter discusses the nature, causes and symptoms of endometriosis as well as aspects such as prevalence, typical age, risk factors and prevention.

When discovered

Endometriosis has probably been around for as long as the human race. The first references to it are believed to be in ancient Egyptian scrolls that date back to 1600BC. However, it was not until 1921 that an American doctor, John Sampson, accurately described the disease and named it endometriosis.

Causes and development

The causes and development of endometriosis are poorly understood despite years of research and speculation. Many theories about the origins and early development have been proposed but it is only in recent years that medical research has become sophisticated enough to start looking at the complex chemical and cellular changes associated with the development of the condition. Hopefully, this research will reveal the answers in the next few years.

Theories of early development

There are four main theories of early development. Each theory is thought to explain how some, but not all, women develop endometriosis.

Retrograde menstruation theory

The theory of retrograde menstruation is by far the most popular theory and it probably explains the vast majority of cases of endometriosis in the pelvic cavity. According to this theory, endometriosis develops when menstrual fluid from the uterus flows backwards through the fallopian tubes and out into the pelvic cavity during the menstrual period. This process of backward flow occurs to some degree in all women with open fallopian tubes and is known as retrograde menstruation.

When the menstrual fluid flows out of the ends of the fallopian tubes it is deposited onto the surrounding organs and tissues. The menstrual fluid contains some of the endometrial cells from the endometrium of the uterus. A number of these cells attach and implant themselves onto the surface of the tissue on which they were deposited and begin to grow and develop into endometrial implants.

Blood and lymph transportation theory

The theory of retrograde menstruation does not explain some of the rare cases where endometrial implants are found outside the pelvic cavity. In these circumstances it would appear that living endometrial cells from the uterine endometrium somehow get into the veins or lymphatic vessels and are transported around the body to another distant site where they implant, grow and develop into endometrial implants.

Accidental transplantation theory

The third theory is that endometriosis can develop by accidental transplantation. In this situation, fragments of endometrium containing endometrial cells are accidentally transported from the uterus to the new site during gynaecological surgery or delivery of a baby. The endometrial cells become lodged in the muscle or tissue at the site of the surgical or caesarian cut and implant themselves in it. The implanted cells then grow and develop into endometrial implants. This theory explains the occasional presence of endometriosis in surgical and caesarian scars. Fortunately, this condition is not common as special precautions are taken to prevent it happening.

Metaplasia theory

According to the metaplasia theory, the peritoneum covering the organs of the pelvic cavity contains primitive cells that were present when the woman herself was an embryo. It is thought that under certain conditions some of these cells are transformed into endometrial cells. The endometrial cells then grow and develop to become endometriosis. It is not known what stimulates the cells to undergo transformation but possible factors are high levels of oestrogen in the pelvic cavity or special chemicals in the retrograde menstrual fluid.

Other factors

None of the endometriosis theories explains the entire process of development. The retrograde menstruation, blood and lymph transportation, and accidental transplantation theories explain how the endometrial cells reach their new sites but they do not explain how and why those cells implant, grow and develop into endometrial implants. Similarly, the metaplasia theory does not explain how and why the primitive cells are transformed into endometrial implants and nodules. Clearly, researchers have unravelled only part of the story.

Much research has been carried out in the last ten years in an attempt to map out the process by which endometriosis develops. Many avenues are being pursued in order to find out what triggers and sustains the development of endometriosis following implantation or metaplasia. Currently, several promising leads are being investigated.

Menstrual and hormonal factors

Traditionally, women spent most of their reproductive years pregnant or breastfeeding a succession of children. Therefore, they had only a few menstrual cycles during their lives. Nowadays, women in our society usually have two or three children at the most so we have more menstrual cycles than earlier generations. As a result, many more endometrial cells are deposited into the pelvic cavity so there are more opportunities for implantation to occur.

The greater number of menstrual cycles experienced by women today means that ovulation occurs more frequently. Ovulation leads to the release of large amounts of oestrogen into the pelvic cavity. Endometriosis seems to need oestrogen to grow and develop. More frequent ovulation means that endometrial implants in the pelvic cavity receive frequent stimulation from oestrogen so they are more likely to survive following implantation.

Immune factors

Part of the immune system consists of a large number of scavenger cells, which are responsible for keeping the pelvic cavity free of unwanted debris. The scavenger cells remove debris such as menstrual fluid by engulfing and digesting it. It is thought that endometriosis may result when there is too much menstrual fluid for the scavenger cells to remove or when there is a problem with the scavenger cell system so that it cannot remove the menstrual fluid as effectively. Either way, not all the menstrual fluid is removed between periods and the excess is left in the pelvic cavity. This may lead to more opportunities for the endometrial cells in the menstrual fluid to implant.

The immune system also comprises a number of chemicals and cells that work together to help protect the pelvic cavity from invasion by foreign matter. Some of these mechanisms do not seem to work well in women with endometriosis. The slightly less effective protection mechanisms may make it easier for the endometrial cells to implant in the pelvic cavity. They may make the peritoneum less resistant to implantation or they may not destroy the retrograde endometrial cells as effectively.

Genetic factors

It seems that some women have a genetic predisposition to developing endometriosis. The pattern of inheritance is not known but it is probably due to the interaction of several genes. The genetic factors may cause a predisposition to developing endometriosis. Alternatively, they may cause the woman to inherit a slightly abnormal immune system that allows easier implantation and growth of the misplaced endometrial cells following retrograde menstruation.

Environmental pollutant factors

Research in the 1980s and early 1990s found that monkeys who were fed small amounts of PCBs and dioxin for several years developed endometriosis. These substances are pollutants that are found in our environment, as well as in our food. Furthermore, the severity of the endometriosis in the monkeys fed dioxin was directly related to the amount of dioxin consumed. In other words, the more dioxin consumed, the more severe the endometriosis.

PCBs and dioxin are known to interfere with the immune system and oestrogen metabolism in animals and humans. When the results of the monkey research became known a few gynaecologists and researchers began to wonder if they could have a role in the development of endometriosis in humans. Several research projects have begun and more are planned. To date there is no conclusive evidence to show whether or not PCBs and dioxin trigger the development of endometriosis in women.

What happens

Once the endometrial cells have implanted they begin to respond to the hormones of the menstrual cycle—in particular, oestrogen and progesterone—in the same way as the endometrium lining the uterus. Thus, the implants grow and swell with blood and then break down and bleed each month. They bleed directly onto the surrounding tissues, which causes irritation and inflammation. The inflammation leads to the development of fibrous tissue around the implant, which may eventually encase it and entrap any future bleeding. Frequently, the irritation and inflammation also cause pain and may lead to the development of adhesions.

Appearance

There are three main forms of endometriosis: endometrial implants, endometrial nodules and endometriomas.

Endometrial implants

Endometrial implants are thought to arise as a result of implantation of endometrial cells from the uterine endometrium. They appear as tiny dots or clusters of dots that lie on the surface of the peritoneum covering the ovaries and the organs of the pelvic cavity. They are usually 1–2 millimetres in diameter and vary in colour from clear or red to black to white depending on their age.

Clear and red implants

Clear and red implants are young implants made up of endometrial cells that have only recently implanted themselves in the pelvic cavity. They are said to be active implants because they undergo regular cycles of growth and bleeding in response to the menstrual hormones. Clear and red implants are often referred to as atypical implants because before the mid-1980s it was not realised that they were a form of endometriosis.

Black implants

Black implants are older implants that have undergone many cycles of growth, bleeding, inflammation and scarring. Over time, some of the old blood that has been shed with each period becomes trapped within the implant giving it a bluish-black appearance. When magnified they may look like clusters of black grapes. They also often have a puckered appearance due to inflammation and scarring around their edges. They are said to be less active implants because they do not undergo such regular cycles of growth and bleeding in response to the menstrual hormones as clear and red implants. Black implants are often referred to as classical implants because for many years they were thought to be the only type of endometrial implant.

White implants

White implants are less well understood. They are probably remnants of old implants that have healed or are inactive.

Microscopic implants

In the early stages of the disease the endometrial implants may be too small to be seen without a microscope. In this situation the implants are sometimes referred to as microscopic endometriosis.

Endometrial nodules

Endometrial nodules are usually found in or near the uterosacral ligaments, the Pouch of Douglas, the cervix, the bowel and the rectovaginal septum. They have a different structure and appearance from implants. They vary in shape but most commonly they are elliptical (elongated) lumps, rather than flat like implants. They are usually 2–3 millimetres in size but may be up to 2 centimetres across. The nodules tend to be white but sometimes there may be a black or yellow-white colouration within them. They are often hard to see because they tend to lie under the peritoneum or infiltrate deep into the underlying tissues. Either the tip of the nodule may be visible or the nodule may be apparent only because it appears as a lump in the overlying surface that may or may not be scarred and puckered. In fact, nodules are often more easily palpated during a pelvic examination (see page 37 in Chapter 3) than seen during a laparoscopy (see pages 69–79 in Chapter 6). They are thought to arise as a result of metaplasia, or growth and infiltration of endometrial implants into the underlying tissue.

Endometriomas

Endometriomas are endometrial cysts that lie within the ovary or on its surface. They are larger than implants and they have an obvious fibrous wall around them. They are usually 4–5 centimetres in diameter but may range from 1–10 centimetres. Endometriomas are sometimes referred to as 'chocolate cysts' because they contain old dark blood that has the appearance and consistency of melted chocolate. There is little consensus about how they arise and develop.

Adhesions

Adhesions are bands of fibrous scar tissue that form inside the body. They vary in appearance from thin, filmy and transparent to thick, dense and opaque. They may be found anywhere in the pelvic area and may extend between almost any combination of organs and tissues. For example, they may bind an ovary to the side of the pelvic cavity, or they may extend between the bladder and the uterus, or they may fix a loop of bowel to the navel—the possibilities are endless. The adhesions themselves may exist as isolated bands or there may be a network of bands that forms a mat over an organ or part of the pelvic cavity. Occasionally, they extend throughout the pelvis creating what is known as a fixed or frozen pelvis.

Adhesions may form as a result of endometrial implants bleeding onto the area around them. The bleeding causes inflammation of the area in the same way that boiling water spilt onto your hand causes inflammation of the skin on your hand. The inflammation leads to the formation of scar tissue as part of the healing process. Unfortunately, in some cases the injured area does not just form a simple scar. Rather, it comes into contact with a nearby inflamed area and forms a band of scar tissue—an adhesion—between the two areas.

Surgery may also lead to the development of adhesions. Many factors associated with surgery can lead to inflammation of the very delicate tissues and organs in the pelvis. The inflammation leads to the formation of adhesions by the same process described above. Adhesions develop within the first three days after surgery and are generally well formed by one to two months. Special surgical techniques have been developed to minimise the formation of adhesions but some women seem susceptible to developing adhesions even with the best techniques.

Sites of endometriosis

The location of endometrial implants depends on how they were transported to their new site. The overwhelming majority of implants are transported to their new location by retrograde menstruation so they are almost always found in the pelvic cavity.

The ovaries are probably the most common site for endometrial implants. The other common sites are the peritoneum, uterosacral ligaments and Pouch of Douglas. These sites lie near and below the ends of the fallopian tubes so they are within the area where most of the retrograde menstrual fluid is deposited. Less common sites include the appendix, surface of the bladder, surface of the uterus, fallopian tubes, surface of the small and large bowels and the rectovaginal septum.

Very rarely, endometrial implants have been found in almost any part of the body, including surgical and caesarian scars, diaphragm, lungs, navel, breasts, arms, legs, groin, nose and eye. These implants are thought to have been transported to the new sites by accidental transplantation (see page 10) or by blood and lymph vessels.

Symptoms of endometriosis

There is a wide range of symptoms that may be associated with endometriosis but the nature and number experienced by individual women varies widely. Some women experience only one or two symptoms, many experience several, and a few unfortunate women experience the full gamut. Some women experience no symptoms and their endometriosis is only discovered during investigations for infertility or during surgery for an unrelated condition. The symptoms experienced by the first 400 women who used the Endometriosis Association (Victoria) Endometriosis Clinic are shown in Table 2.1.

The key feature of most endometriosis symptoms is that they are cyclical. In other words, they vary in intensity with the menstrual cycle. The symptoms are usually present or are worse around the time of ovulation or menstruation.

The severity of symptoms varies from mild to severe but it is not necessarily related to the severity of the disease. Mild endometriosis may cause severe pain while severe disease may cause moderate pain. The severity of a symptom depends more on the location of the implants causing the symptom. One or two implants or nodules in the Pouch of Douglas, uterosacral ligaments or rectovaginal septum

Table 2.1   Symptoms of endometriosis

Symptom	Percentage of women who experienced the symptom
Dysmenorrhoea (painful periods)	82
Pelvic pain	66
Dyspareunia (painful intercourse)	60
Bloating	59
Lower back pain	57
Ovulation pain	54
Constipation and/or diarrhoea	52
Fatigue	51
Rectal pain	44
Heavy bleeding	42
Painful bowel movements	38
Premenstrual spotting	31
Frequent urination	31
Infertility	17
Pain when urinating	16

may cause excruciating pain, whereas a sprinkling of implants on the peritoneum may cause much less pain.

The range and severity of symptoms often increases as the disease progresses. In addition, the number of days in the month for which the symptoms are felt often increases as the condition worsens. These changes are usually insidious. In the early stages of the disease the symptoms may be mild and apparent for only the first one or two days of a period but as the condition worsens the symptoms may be felt with increasing severity for more days of the month. For some women, however, the number and severity of their symptoms remains constant for many years.

Dysmenorrhoea (period pain)

Dysmenorrhoea means painful periods and it is the most common symptom of endometriosis. Many women experience intense pain during their periods, necessitating time at home in bed with hot water bottles and analgesics.

According to medical textbooks there are two types of dysmenorrhoea: primary and secondary. Primary dysmenorrhoea is said to be the 'cramping' type of dysmenorrhoea that typically affects teenagers. It usually begins a year or two after the onset of menstruation and tends to diminish by the age of 25 or after childbirth. The pain usually begins with the menstrual flow and lasts for one or two days. It is often accompanied by nausea, vomiting, diarrhoea, dizziness and fainting. This type of dysmenorrhoea is generally believed to have no relationship to endometriosis. Secondary dysmenorrhoea is menstrual pain that is a result of an underlying condition of the reproductive organs. This type of dysmenorrhoea is generally believed to be associated with conditions such as endometriosis.

The pain of dysmenorrhoea caused by endometriosis may be mild, moderate or severe. It has been described by women as constant, deep inside, sharp, stabbing, knife-like, nagging, aching, burning, throbbing, dull, boring and cramping. It may be located in the centre or on one or both sides of the abdomen. The pain may radiate into the vulva, pubic bone, lower back, rectum, buttocks, groin and thighs. The pain may begin one to several days before the start of the period and gradually become more severe, particularly once the menstrual flow begins. It may last for the first one to two days of the period or continue throughout the period. Usually, the pain is most severe on the first or second day of the period.

What causes the dysmenorrhoea associated with endometriosis is not known precisely but it is probably due to several reasons. One reason is that the bleeding from the endometrial implants causes irritation to and inflammation of the surrounding tissues. This in turn leads to the release of pain-producing chemicals known as prostaglandins (see page 103, in Chapter 8). Another possible reason is that bleeding into the older implants and nodules causes pressure and hence pain in much the same way that a boil causes pain.

Dyspareunia (painful sexual intercourse)

Dyspareunia is a very common but often unacknowledged symptom of endometriosis. This symptom causes much heartache for women with endometriosis and it can have a devastating effect on their self-esteem and sexual relationships. More information on coping with dyspareunia can be found on pages 162–4 in Chapter 13.

Dyspareunia caused by endometriosis may be felt during intercourse or for up to 24–48 hours after intercourse or both. In some cases it may just cause discomfort but often the symptom is so severe that it makes intercourse impossible. The pain may be described as sharp, stabbing, jabbing or a deep ache. Intercourse may always cause pain, or it may cause pain only at certain times of the month, such as during menstruation or at ovulation. The pain may be felt only with deep penetration or it may be felt with any form of intercourse.

Dyspareunia is usually associated with implants and nodules in the Pouch of Douglas, the uterosacral ligaments or the rectovaginal septum. It may also be associated with implants on the vagina or cervix. If the implants or nodules are located in the Pouch of Douglas, the uterosacral ligaments or the rectovaginal septum, the pain may be due to stretching and pulling of the implants and nodules in those tissues.

Pain during vaginal examinations

Some women with endometriosis experience pain during vaginal examinations. The pain experienced is similar to that experienced with intercourse and is the result of irritation from implants and nodules in the Pouch of Douglas, the uterosacral ligaments and the rectovaginal septum.

Pelvic pain

Some women experience pelvic pain that is not associated with their periods. Pelvic pain can be soul destroying because trying to cope with pain day in and day out is extremely tiring and depressing, especially if it is unrelenting.

Pelvic pain may be experienced constantly or intermittently. If the pain is intermittent it may be unpredictable and come and go during the day or from day to day. Alternatively, it may be provoked by certain positions, such as sitting, and certain movements, such as reaching up or jogging. The nature of the pain varies widely but it has been described as a dragging or pulling sensation, a constant dull ache, or a throb. The intensity tends to vary over time so that sometimes the pain is manageable and at other times it is not. The pain may be generalised throughout the pelvic area, or it may affect one side of the pelvic area, or it may be localised to one particular site. Pelvic pain may be caused by tension on endometrial implants and nodules, pressure from an endometrioma, or adhesions pulling on organs.

Lower back pain

Lower back pain is a far more common symptom of endometriosis than is generally realised. It can be a very tiring symptom because it tends to be unrelenting. The pain may range from mild to debilitating and it is usually described as a deep ache. It may be felt at ovulation, up to a week before menstruation, during menstruation, or throughout the month. Lower back pain is usually due to irritation from implants and nodules in the Pouch of Douglas, the uterosacral ligaments and the rectovaginal septum.

Ovulation pain

Many women without endometriosis experience some discomfort at the time of ovulation. However, the ovulation pain experienced by women with endometriosis tends to be more severe and often lasts much longer. The pain may precede ovulation by 12–24 hours and it may last for 4–5 days. Ovulation pain is usually felt only on one side—over the ovary that is ovulating that month—but sometimes it is felt on both sides. The pain is probably due to slight enlargement of the ovary at the time of ovulation. The enlargement stretches endometrial implants on the ovary, compresses and stretches endometriomas, and stretches adhesions on the surface of the ovary.

Bowel symptoms

Bowel symptoms are among the least recognised symptoms of endometriosis but they can play havoc with women's lives. Although the bowel is not part of the reproductive system, the lower end of the bowel lies adjacent to the areas most commonly affected by endometrial implants and nodules. Because the connection between bowel symptoms and endometriosis is often overlooked, many women have considerable difficulty having their symptoms recognised as being associated with their endometriosis.

Most bowel symptoms are not caused by the presence of endometriosis on the surface of the bowel itself. Rather, they are usually the result of irritation from implants and nodules located in adjacent areas such as the Pouch of Douglas, the uterosacral ligaments or the rectovaginal septum. Sometimes, they may be caused by adhesions constricting or pulling on the bowel. The range of bowel symptoms varies. The most common are diarrhoea, constipation, alternating bouts of constipation and diarrhoea, painful bowel movements, rectal pain, pain when passing wind, abdominal bloating, pain during rectal examinations, abdominal pain, cramps, spasms, nausea and vomiting. These symptoms are more commonly felt at the time of menstruation although they may be present throughout the month.

In those cases where the endometrial implants are located on the bowel, the implants are usually lying on the outside of the bowel wall rather than in the bowel itself. The symptoms experienced in this situation are the same as those experienced when the nodules are located in adjacent areas. If implants are located in the bowel wall rectal bleeding may be experienced in addition to the symptoms listed above.

Bladder symptoms

Implants on or in the bladder wall, or irritation from implants on organs and tissues that lie against the bladder, such as the front of the uterus, may cause a range of bladder symptoms. The most common are pain in the bladder region, pain or burning when urinating, frequent urination and blood in the urine. These symptoms are more commonly felt at the time of menstruation although they may be present throughout the month.

Bleeding symptoms

The most common bleeding problems associated with endo-metriosis are heavy bleeding, clotting and premenstrual spotting. Heavy bleeding with or without clotting is a common symptom. There is much debate about what constitutes heavy bleeding. However, it would seem rea-sonable to assume that any woman can be said to have heavy bleeding if it interferes with her normal lifestyle. Premenstrual spotting is spotting or staining that occurs for more than 12–24 hours before the onset of the period. The spotting is usually a brownish colour. It is not known what causes the bleeding symptoms but it is possible that they are due to hormonal disturbances.

Abdominal bloating

Abdominal bloating is a common but rarely recognised symptom of endometriosis and it is the bane of many women's lives. Women often say that abdominal bloating makes them look about four months pregnant and some even have to keep two sets of clothes—the larger set being for when they are bloated. The bloating may be present most of the time, at ovulation, for a week or so before menstruation, or during menstruation. No-one really knows what causes the bloating but it may be the result of the inflammation associated with endometriosis or it may be the result of irritation to the bowel.

Fatigue

Fatigue is a common but largely unrecognised symptom of endometriosis. Most women with endometriosis suffer some fatigue but for a few it is their main symptom. In milder cases the fatigue may mean that the woman has trouble getting through the day and does not have the energy to go out and socialise. In more severe cases it may be so debilitating that she is unable to hold down a job or look after her family adequately. The fatigue is probably a result of pain, and the inflammation and other disease processes associated with endometriosis.

Adhesions

Most adhesions do not cause symptoms but the few that do can cause havoc. In some cases, they cause more problems than the endometriosis itself.

The symptoms of adhesions are often similar to those of endometriosis. As a result, they are often confused with each other. Adhesions can cause a wide variety of symptoms, including dyspareunia, localised or generalised pelvic pain, ovulation pain, bowel symptoms and bladder symptoms. The symptoms experienced will depend on the site of the adhesions. For example, an ovary stuck to the side of the pelvis may cause localised pelvic pain and ovulation pain. Adhesions on the bowel may fix it to other organs that restrict its movement and lead to bowel symptoms. Severe scarring and adhesions encircling and constricting the bowel may lead to an obstruction of the bowel.

Adhesions can cause pain ranging in intensity from mild to incapacitating. Because adhesions are a consequence of endometriosis they do not change cyclically with the menstrual cycle like the true symptoms of endometriosis. Therefore, the pain is often present for much of the time although the intensity usually varies. In some cases, the pain is felt during and after activities that stretch the adhesions, such as exercise, intercourse or internal examinations. This pain may take several hours or days to subside.

Infertility

Infertility is one of the most well-recognised symptoms of endometriosis although it is less common than many of the other symptoms. Information on infertility can be found on pages 115–18 in Chapter 9.

Progression

No-one really knows how endometriosis progresses if left untreated. To get an overall picture of the way the disease progresses researchers would need to do laparoscopies at regular intervals on thousands of untreated women for many years—something that cannot be justified.

Many gynaecologists presume that endometriosis is a progressive condition. In other words, they believe that it is a condition that, if left untreated, will progressively worsen in extent and severity until the woman's oestrogen levels fall with the onset of the menopause. However, there is increasing evidence that many cases of endometriosis are stable or resolving spontaneously. This appears to be especially so for women with minimal or mild endometriosis.

Among those women whose disease is progressive, the rate of progression varies widely. For most, it is fairly slow and the disease gradually worsens over a number of years. However, it appears that in a few women the disease progresses rapidly and, in some cases, the progression may be so rapid that their endometriosis goes from mild to severe in a matter of months. Unfortunately, it is impossible to predict the likely rate of progression in any particular woman.

Prevalence

Because very little research has been done investigating its prevalence, the true frequency of endometriosis in the community is not known. Even if such studies were undertaken it would be very difficult to determine the true figure because many women are undiagnosed. Nevertheless, gynaecologists generally say that endometriosis affects about 10 per cent of women at some stage during their menstruating years. The only reasonably reliable study that has attempted to estimate the prevalence is a study in the United States which found that about 3 per cent of women in the subject community had endometriosis.

There is much debate as to whether or not endometriosis is becoming more common. Some gynaecologists believe there has been an increase in the number of women who have endometriosis—and that the condition has become more common—because women are having fewer children and having them later in life. A few gynaecologists also believe that the disease is becoming more common due to the increasing presence of pollutants such as PCBs and dioxin in our environment.

Alternatively, other gynaecologists believe that there has only been an increase in the number of women being diagnosed. They believe that a greater proportion of women are now being diagnosed because there is better awareness and recognition of the condition by the medical profession and because access to laparoscopy has made it much easier to diagnose the condition.

Typical age

Endometriosis usually affects women only during their menstruating years—it does not occur before the onset of menstruation and it is rarely found after the menopause. However, the true age distribution of endometriosis is not known because the relevant research has not been done.

Before the introduction of laparoscopy in the 1970s most gynaecologists believed that endometriosis was a condition of women in their thirties and forties. When laparoscopy became a standard part of the infertility investigation it became apparent that many women undergoing investigation had endometriosis. These women were primarily women in their late twenties and early thirties. Gynaecologists then accepted the view that endometriosis was most commonly found in women in that age group. Furthermore, they believed that endometriosis was uncommon in young women under the age of 25 and rare in teenagers.

Research conducted in the 1980s by the Endometriosis Association (Victoria) and the North American-based Endometriosis Association found that, although most women with endometriosis were being diagnosed in their late twenties and early thirties, many women had had their endometriosis symptoms since their teenage years. Their endometriosis had not been diagnosed earlier because their doctors had not considered it before the women reached the typical age range for endometriosis.

As a result of the research, it is now being increasingly realised that endometriosis is more common in teenagers and young women under the age of 25 than was previously thought. Consequently, more teenagers and young women with symptoms of endometriosis are being investigated and diagnosed while the disease is still in its early stages. Hopefully, this trend will continue as more doctors become aware of the possibility of endometriosis in teenagers and young women.

Risk factors

Research aimed at discovering the factors that increase or decrease a woman's risk of developing endometriosis has been conducted only in recent years. Many of the results obtained have been contradictory. Nevertheless, several avenues seem promising and research is continuing.

Considerable attention is being devoted to investigating factors that lead to a greater amount of retrograde menstrual flow and hence a greater likelihood of endometriosis. Potential factors include starting menstruation at an early age, short menstrual cycles, long periods, heavy bleeding, use of an intra-uterine device (IUD) and not bearing any children. Factors that are likely to decrease the amount of menstrual flow and hence decrease the likelihood of endo-metriosis are also being investigated. The factor most commonly investigated in this context has been use of the oral contraceptive pill as the pill usually results in lighter periods.

Research is also focusing on factors that may result in lower oestrogen levels in the body as it is thought that endometriosis is less likely to develop if oestrogen levels are lower. The main potential risk factor being investigated here is regular vigorous exercise because exercise usually leads to a reduction in oestrogen levels.

The risk factor that has shown the clearest results to date is inheritance. It seems that having a mother or sister with endometriosis increases the likelihood of developing the condition by six to nine times. The pattern of inheritance is not known but it is likely that several genes are involved and that the mechanisms by which the genes trigger the development of endometriosis are complex.

Prevention

Gynaecologists and researchers have not been able to find a way of preventing endometriosis because as yet no-one knows what causes it, what factors trigger and sustain its development, or who is most at risk of developing the condition.

Much research is being carried out in order to ascertain the risk factors for endometriosis. It is hoped that in the future it may be possible to identify those women and girls who are most at risk of developing the condition. It may then be possible to offer them advice regarding what they could do to reduce their risk of developing the disease.

Eventually, when more is known about what determines how and why endometrial implants develop in some women and not others, it may be possible to find ways to prevent endometriosis occurring or at least to prevent recurrences of the condition. For example, it may be possible to develop a vaccine against the condition or to design drugs that cure it permanently.

Endometriosis and cancer

Over the years the finding of cancers in some women with endometriosis has led to speculation about the possibility that women with endometriosis may be more at risk of developing cancer. Unfortunately, a recent study has indicated that this may be so. A comprehensive study conducted in Sweden has found that women with endometriosis are 20 per cent more likely to develop cancer than women without.

The study found that women with endometriosis are nearly twice as likely to develop ovarian cancer as women in the general community. This equates to a 1.9 per cent chance compared with a 1.0 per cent chance for women in the general community. However, this risk is still low. The risk was higher in women with a long-standing history of ovarian endometriosis. Women with endometriosis were also 30 per cent more likely to develop breast cancer. This represents a 10.8 per cent chance compared with an 8.3 per cent chance for women in the general population. The reasons for the higher risks of ovarian and breast cancer are not understood but they could be linked to the lower rate of childbearing in women with endometriosis because having no children is known to increase the risk of these two cancers.

The researchers found that the rates of cervical cancer and endometrial cancer in women with endometriosis were the same as for women in the general community.

Surprisingly, the research also showed an increased rate of non-Hodgkin's lymphoma, which is a cancer of the lymph tissue. This cancer was found to be 80 per cent more common in women with endometriosis. This equates to a 2.1 per cent chance compared with a 1.2 per cent chance for women in general, which is still a low risk.

These findings come from only one study so further research is needed before we can verify their accuracy. Nevertheless, in the meantime, women with endometriosis should be aware that they may have an increased risk of developing some cancers and they should discuss the need for ongoing monitoring with their doctor.

3
Diagnosis of endometriosis

There is no simple test that can be used to detect endometriosis. The only reliable way to diagnose the condition is by observing the endometrial implants, nodules and endometriomas during an operation known as a laparoscopy.

A diagnosis usually involves several stages that will include some or all of the following:

- reporting your symptoms
- giving a history of your symptoms
- having a physical examination
- having an ultrasound
- having a laparoscopy.

Unfortunately, for many women the road to diagnosis takes years rather than months and it is not uncommon for women to see several doctors regarding their symptoms before a diagnosis is made. This long delay in diagnosis is partly due to the fact that endometriosis can be difficult to diagnose. The symptoms are similar to those of several other conditions so women are sometimes diagnosed with those conditions rather than with endometriosis. The delay is also due to many GPs' lack of knowledge of the symptoms of endometriosis. Research by the Endometriosis Association (Victoria) ('the Association') found that most GPs recognised only four of the common symptoms and were not aware of the wide range of other possible symptoms. In addition, GPs have been taught that endometriosis is a condition of women in their late twenties and early thirties. Research by the Association indicates that many women are being diagnosed in their late twenties and early thirties despite reporting symptoms for many years previously, because that is the age when their doctors initially consider a diagnosis of endometriosis and carry out the necessary investigations.

This chapter discusses the diagnosis of endometriosis and the conditions that are commonly confused with endometriosis.

Reporting your symptoms

The first stage along the road to a diagnosis of endometriosis is reporting your symptoms to a GP or gynaecologist. This is often not an easy step as it involves acknowledging that you have symptoms that are causing major difficulties or that need investigating or both. Research by the Association has shown that it takes women an average of 1.6 years after the onset of symptoms to make this step.

If you suspect that you may have endometriosis you should report your symptoms to a doctor as soon as possible. Early diagnosis and treatment may reduce the likelihood of long-term complications such as chronic pain and adhesions. You may reasonably suspect endometriosis if you have some of the following symptoms:

* dysmenorrhoea (painful periods)
* dyspareunia (painful intercourse)
* pelvic pain (not necessarily at the time of your period)
* lower back pain
* ovulation pain
* bowel symptoms (especially at the time of your period)
* heavy bleeding.

You may especially suspect endometriosis if your symptoms are:

* so painful or severe that you have to take time off work
* so painful that you have to stay in bed
* not helped by taking painkillers such as Panadol

- not helped by taking non-steroidal anti-inflammatory drugs such as Ponstan and Naprogesic
- not helped by taking the oral contraceptive pill
- occurring at the same time every month
- gradually getting worse.

You may need to report your symptoms to your GP several times before he or she considers a diagnosis of endometriosis and refers you to a gynaecologist. It may help to suggest a diagnosis of endometriosis as many GPs do not think of it until all other diagnoses have been eliminated. Be persistent and do whatever is needed to have your symptoms properly investigated. Remember that you can request a referral to a gynaecologist.

Giving a history

A diagnosis of endometriosis cannot be made on the basis of the history of your symptoms alone but it is an essential guide for the gynaecologist. Information about your symptoms gives the gynaecologist an indication of the likelihood that you have endometriosis. If your history suggests that you may have endometriosis, your gynaecologist will recommend that you have a laparoscopy to confirm the diagnosis.

Taking a history for endometriosis involves building up a detailed picture of the nature and occurrence of your symptoms. In order to maximise your chances of being diagnosed it is important that you give your gynaecologist as comprehensive a history as possible of all your symptoms. You should outline the nature, onset, timing, severity and progression of all your symptoms, even if discussing a particular symptom such as painful intercourse is embarrassing. It may be worthwhile preparing a concise summary of your symptoms and their history before your visit to the gynaecologist. You could either give the summary to the gynaecologist to read or use it as a checklist when talking about your symptoms.

On your first visit to the gynaecologist you will be asked many questions about your periods, pain and other symptoms. If the gynaecologist does not ask any questions about an aspect of your symptoms that you think is important, make sure that you mention it. Below is a list of some of the questions the gynaecologist may ask.

Periods

- How old were you when your periods started?
- When was your last period?
- Are your periods regular?
- How long do your periods last?
- How heavy are your periods (i.e., how many pads and/or tampons do you use each period)?
- Do you pass clots or have flooding during your periods?
- Do you have a brownish discharge before your period starts?
- Do you have any bleeding or spotting between your periods?

Period pain

- Do you have pain with your periods?
- When did you start having painful periods?
- Do you have pain before your period starts?
- Do you have pain for the first day only of your period?
- Do you have pain throughout your period?
- For how many hours or days does your period pain last?
- Where do you feel your period pain?
- Can you describe your period pain?
- Is your period pain gradually getting worse?
- Is your period pain accompanied by sweating, nausea, vomiting, constipation or diarrhoea?
- Does your period pain wake you up at night?

- Is your period pain severe enough to restrict your normal activities? If so, how?
- Do you have to stay in bed when you have period pain?
- Are there any measures that help relieve your period pain?
- Do you need to take painkilling tablets for your period pain? If so, what do you take and does it relieve the pain?

Other pain

- Do you have pain during or after intercourse?
- Do you have pain when passing urine or using your bowels?
- Do you have pain at ovulation?
- Do you have pelvic pain other than period pain or ovulation pain?
- Can you describe the pain you experience?
- When do you experience these symptoms?
- Is your pain severe enough to restrict your normal activities? If so, how?
- Do you have to stay in bed when you have pain?
- What makes your pain better or worse?
- Do you need to take painkilling tablets for your pain? If so, what do you take and does it relieve the pain?

Other symptoms

- Do you have constipation and/or diarrhoea?
- Do you have lower back pain or leg pain?
- Do you suffer from chronic fatigue?
- Do you suffer from migraine?
- When do you experience these symptoms?
- Have you ever tried to conceive or have you been having unprotected intercourse? If so, for how long?
- Have your mother or sister had period pain or endometriosis?

Having a physical examination

A physical examination usually involves an examination of your breasts and abdomen, and a pelvic examination (sometimes also known as an internal or a vaginal examination). A pelvic examination is an examination in which the gynaecologist feels and palpates the reproductive organs. The purpose of the examination is to try to ascertain whether you may have endometriosis. If you have not had a pelvic examination before, ask the gynaecologist to explain the procedure. Knowing what is involved will help you relax. This will make the examination more comfortable for you and easier for the gynaecologist.

A pelvic examination may cause discomfort but it should not be painful. If the examination causes any discomfort or pain, tell the gynaecologist and if necessary ask him or her to stop for a moment to allow the pain to subside.

A pelvic examination can only give an indication that you may have endometriosis. If the gynaecologist is able to feel tender nodules in the Pouch of Douglas area, the likelihood that you have endometriosis is increased. If the ovary feels enlarged there is a possibility that you may have a cyst, such as an endometrioma. Usually, however, nothing abnormal will be found as endometrial implants are too small for the gynaecologist to feel during a pelvic examination.

Having an ultrasound

Ultrasound involves the use of high-frequency sound waves to create a picture of the body. Over the last decade vaginal ultrasound has been used increasingly to help diagnose endometriosis. A vaginal ultrasound is one where the probe is inserted into the vagina rather than moved over the abdomen. It results in a clearer picture of the ovaries and uterus than is possible with an abdominal ultrasound.

Vaginal ultrasound is sometimes a useful adjunct in the diagnosis of endometriosis as it can detect endometriomas lying on or within the ovary. This enables the gynaecologist to determine the size and location of the endometrioma so that the surgery to remove it can be planned accordingly. Vaginal ultrasound is especially useful if the endometrioma lies within the ovary as it is not always possible to see such endometriomas during surgery. It can also ascertain if an ovary is bound down by adhesions. This will tell your gynaecologist that you have adhesions that need to be cut during your laparoscopy.

Ultrasound should not be used as a substitute for laparoscopy. It cannot detect endometrial implants so it cannot diagnose most cases of endometriosis. A normal ultrasound does not mean that you do not have endometriosis—women with severe endometriosis often have a normal ultrasound.

One of the main benefits of vaginal ultrasound is its ability to detect some conditions that have similar symptoms to endometriosis and which are often confused with it. Polycystic ovaries and adenomyosis are two conditions that are commonly confused with endometriosis and which can usually be detected using a vaginal ultrasound (see pages 40–1).

Having a laparoscopy

Even if your history, pelvic examination and ultrasound strongly suggest that you have endometriosis, you must have an operation known as a laparoscopy to confirm the diagnosis. Endometriosis is easily confused with several other conditions so it is essential that the gynaecologist inspects your pelvic cavity to ascertain whether you have endometriosis or another condition. A laparoscopy is the most effective way of inspecting the pelvic cavity for signs of the condition.

A laparoscopy also enables the gynaecologist to accurately assess the location, extent and severity of your endometriosis. You and your gynaecologist will need this information to make decisions about your treatment.

Information about having a laparoscopy can be found on pages 69–79 in Chapter 6. Details of what the gynaecologist will be looking for during the inspection of your pelvis and what surgical procedures can be done at the time of diagnosis are also included.

During the laparoscopy the gynaecologist will probably remove a few samples of suspected endometrial implants to send to the pathologist. These will be carefully inspected under the microscope to confirm the diagnosis.

Classifying endometriosis

There are a number of ways of classifying the severity of endometriosis using a formal scoring system. The most commonly used system assigns different scores to the various types of endometriosis and adds up all the scores. For example, an endometrial implant may be given a score of 1 and an endometrioma a larger score. The total score is then used to classify the woman's endometriosis.

Few gynaecologists in Australia use such scoring systems. Most classify the severity of the disease according to their visual impression during a laparoscopy. The categories most commonly used are minimal, mild, moderate and severe. The terms stage I, stage II, stage III and stage IV are also used. The terms may be used interchangeably, as stage I corresponds to minimal disease, stage II to mild disease, and so on.

It is important to remember that the classification system rates the severity of your endometriosis only according to the number and size of any implants, nodules, endometriomas and adhesions present. It does not necessarily bear any relationship to the severity of your symptoms.

Minimal or mild endometriosis can cause severe symptoms while severe endometriosis may cause mild symptoms.

Conditions confused with endometriosis

Some of the symptoms of endometriosis are also the symptoms of a number of other conditions, so endometriosis is sometimes confused with them. These conditions include irritable bowel syndrome, polycystic ovaries, adenomyosis, ovarian cysts, pelvic inflammatory disease, appendicitis and cancer.

Irritable bowel syndrome

Irritable bowel syndrome is a term used to describe a variety of bowel symptoms when no other diagnosis can be found. The symptoms include lower abdominal pain that may or may not be relieved by bowel movements, bouts of diarrhoea and constipation, wind, straining to open the bowels, bloated abdomen, back pain, lethargy, nausea and heartburn. Many women are diagnosed as having irritable bowel syndrome before ultimately being diagnosed with endometriosis.

Polycystic ovaries

Polycystic ovaries, or PCO as they are often called, are ovaries that contain an excessive number of follicles (see page 2 in Chapter 1). Normal ovaries contain 5–10 follicles, but in polcystic ovaries the ovary contains at least 15 and occasionally as many as 30–50 follicles. Polycystic ovaries can cause pelvic pain. If the polycystic ovaries cause other symptoms the condition is referred to as polycystic ovarian syndrome, or PCOS. The symptoms that may be experienced with PCOS are weight gain, infrequent or irregular periods, excessive hair growth, acne and infertility.

Adenomyosis

Adenomyosis is a condition in which endometrium is found in the myometrium of the uterus (see page 1 in Chapter 1). The extent of the adenomyosis varies: it may be restricted to a small area or it may extend through much of the uterus. It is most commonly found in women between the ages of 40 and 50. The main symptoms are heavy bleeding, painful periods and irregular bleeding, although about a third of women with adenomyosis have no symptoms.

Ovarian cysts

A cyst is a growth that contains fluid and is enclosed by a membrane. There are many types of ovarian cysts. The symptoms that may be experienced with ovarian cysts include abdominal pain on the affected side; pain with intercourse; abdominal swelling, fullness or discomfort; and irregularities of the menstrual cycle. If the cyst is large it may put pressure on adjacent organs, such as the bowel and bladder, which may in turn cause discomfort with bowel movements or when passing urine.

Pelvic inflammatory disease

Pelvic inflammatory disease, often known as PID, is an infection of the pelvic organs. The infection may involve the ovaries, fallopian tubes, uterus or cervix. The symptoms may include painful periods, pain during or after inter-course, bleeding between periods, painful bowel move-ments, generalised pelvic pain, lower back pain, nausea, fatigue, low-grade fever and infertility.

Acute appendicitis

Acute appendicitis is an inflammation of the appendix. The symptoms include sudden and severe right-sided abdominal pain, nausea and vomiting, malaise and a raised temperature. The symptoms of acute appendicitis are sometimes confused with the rupture of a large endometrioma.

Cancer

Cancers are rarely confused with endometriosis. If there is any possibility that you may have cancer the appropriate tests will be carried out immediately. The two main forms of cancer that could possibly be confused with endometriosis are ovarian cancer and rectal cancer. The symptoms of ovarian cancer may include pelvic pain, weight loss, weakness and anaemia. The symptoms of rectal cancer may include constipation, bleeding from the rectum and back pain.

4
Treatment overview

No single treatment for endometriosis has been developed that is effective for all women. A vast array of approaches has been tried, each of which is effective for some women. This chapter outlines the wide range of treatments available for endometriosis and discusses a number of the circumstances that may influence your choice of treatments.

Forms of treatment

The main forms of treatment for endometriosis are:

- monitoring
- symptomatic management
- hormonal treatment
- surgical treatment
- self-help and complementary therapies
- combined treatment.

Monitoring

Monitoring involves no active treatment. Rather, it involves regular visits to the gynaecologist to review your symptoms and general wellbeing.

Monitoring is most commonly used after hormonal or surgical treatment to watch for the return of symptoms as this is seen to be a sign that your endometriosis is recurring. Monitoring may also be used after a diagnostic laparoscopy if you decide not to have treatment. Sometimes monitoring is recommended for women with mild disease because the gynaecologist feels that their symptoms are not severe enough to warrant treatment at this stage.

Symptomatic management

The symptomatic management of endometriosis involves treating only the symptoms rather than the underlying disease. It usually involves treating the pain associated with endometriosis using analgesic or non-steroidal anti-inflammatory drugs (see pages 104–8 in Chapter 8).

Symptomatic management is mainly used to help manage the pain associated with chronic endometriosis that has not been successfully treated with hormonal or surgical treatment, or when the woman wants a break from treatment. It is also used to treat the pain associated with adhesions. Sometimes, symptomatic management is used as an adjunct to hormonal or complementary therapies to relieve the symptoms before the treatment begins to be effective.

If you decide to have only this form of treatment, you must be aware that your endometriosis will not be treated in any way and that it may worsen.

Hormonal treatment

The hormonal treatment of endometriosis uses a variety of drugs to treat the condition. In general, hormonal treatments aim to eradicate the endometriosis by suppressing the menstrual cycle and preventing the growth and development of endometrial implants.

Surgical treatment

The surgical treatment of endometriosis aims to remove as many endometrial implants, nodules, endometriomas and adhesions as possible, and to repair any damage caused by the disease.

Self-help and complementary therapies

Self-help therapies aim to improve your overall health and wellbeing and hence your body's ability to heal itself. Complementary therapists use a wide range of therapies to treat women with endometriosis. The treatment used will depend on the therapist's assessment of your condition, plus his or her expertise and preferences as well as your preferences.

Combined treatment

Combined treatment is the concurrent use of two forms of treatment. It is usually done to try to eradicate chronic endometriosis, or to help control symptoms during or after treatment. Most commonly, it involves surgery followed by hormonal treatment, or simultaneous hormonal treatment and complementary therapies, or surgery followed by symptomatic management.

Treatment options

The forms of treatment used by women often change over time. Women with easily treated endometriosis may only ever need one course of treatment. However, women with recurrent or chronic endometriosis may try several different forms of treatment during their lives.

Most newly diagnosed women will have either hormonal or surgical treatment as their first course of treatment. In the past, most women were given a course of hormonal treatment following diagnosis. Nowadays, however, a greater proportion are having surgical treatment at the time of diagnosis.

In the past, women with multiple recurrences of their endometriosis usually tried a succession of surgical and hormonal treatments. At some stage many experimented with one or more complementary therapies to replace or augment their hormonal and surgical treatments. Now, with greater acceptability and availability of complementary therapies, many women are experimenting with complementary therapies soon after diagnosis.

Not only are there several different forms of treatment, but within each category there are a number of possible treatments. The range of options for treating your endometriosis is vast. If you want to take an active role in managing your endometriosis, you need to spend time reading and thinking about the options that might suit you. The next four chapters discuss in detail the options readily available in Australia.

Choosing treatments

In general, you can select from the full range of treatment options but there are several situations when endometriosis can only be treated surgically. Endometrial nodules, endometriomas and adhesions can only be removed surgically as hormonal treatment has no long-term effect on them. Similarly, if your endometriosis has caused damage to any organs in the pelvic cavity, the damage can only be repaired surgically.

Deciding which treatment to use can be daunting. Give yourself enough time to research the information and think about the possibilities before making your final decision.

Hormonal treatment

Some women choose hormonal treatment rather than surgery because they feel it is a less drastic form of treatment. Others do not want to have to take time off for surgery, while others simply do not like the idea of having surgery. Some women, particularly those who have previously developed severe adhesions following surgery, choose hormonal treatment because they do not want to take the risk of developing further adhesions. And some women choose hormonal treatment because they cannot afford the cost of surgery.

Surgical treatment

Women sometimes choose surgical treatment rather than hormonal treatment because they have heard stories about the possible side effects associated with hormonal treatment or they themselves have experienced intolerable side effects on hormonal treatment. Others choose surgery because they are concerned about the possible long-term side effects of using drugs for extended periods. Some simply do not like the idea of taking drugs. And some women choose surgery because they do not want to delay trying to get pregnant for another 6 to 9 months while they undergo hormonal treatment.

Complementary therapies

Choosing which complementary therapies to use is a matter of personal preference as there has been almost no research comparing their effectiveness for endometriosis. Furthermore, each therapist has a favoured way of treating the condition. You need to choose a therapy that seems 'right' for you and to find a practitioner whose approach and manner you feel comfortable with.

Effectiveness

No treatment for endometriosis offers a magical or permanent cure. Although success rates for some treatments have been published, it is not possible to predict the likelihood of your treatment being successful. In general, gynaecologists believe that the milder your endometriosis, the more likely that your treatment will be successful. Conversely, they also believe that the more severe your endometriosis, the less likely the treatment will be successful. However, there is a wide variation in the way women respond to the various treatments so it is not possible to predict how you will respond to any treatment.

Recurrence

Regardless of the type of treatment used, some women will have a recurrence of their symptoms. Studies indicate that approximately 20 per cent of women will have a recurrence within 12 months and as many as 50 per cent within five years. Most gynaecologists believe that women with severe endometriosis are more likely to have a recurrence of their symptoms than women with a milder form of the disease, and that they are likely to have a recurrence sooner.

It is not known what causes recurrences of endometriosis following treatment. It may be due to the regrowth of implants and nodules that were not completely eradicated during treatment, or the deposition and implantation of new endometrial cells in the pelvic cavity and their subsequent growth and development into endometrial implants. It may also be due to a combination of both mechanisms.

5
Hormonal treatments

There are ten hormonal drugs that are commonly used to manage endometriosis in Australia. They fall into four main groups: the pill, the progesterone-like drugs, the androgenic-like drugs, and the GnRH agonists.

The types of the pill commonly used for endometriosis include Brevinor, Brevinor–1 and Norinyl–1. They are not commonly used nowadays to eradicate active endometriosis. Rather, they are more often used to prevent endometriosis developing or getting worse. The side effects are the same as those experienced when using the pill as a contraceptive.

The progesterone-like drugs are usually referred to as the progestogens. They include Provera, Duphaston and Depo-Provera. The side effects experienced tend to be those commonly associated with premenstrual syndrome (PMS). Most women will experience at least one or two manageable side effects.

The androgenic-like drugs are danazol and Dimetriose. Both drugs can be associated with a wide range of side effects, although the number and severity experienced by individual women varies widely.

The two GnRH agonists available in Australia are Synarel and Zoladex. The vast majority of women will experience menopausal-type side effects, but most women will find them tolerable.

Although no one drug is 100 per cent effective on all women, there are no significant differences in the effectiveness of the drugs that have been tested in clinical trials. Provera, danazol, Dimetriose, Synarel and Zoladex are all equally effective in treating the pain symptoms of endometriosis and eradicating endometrial implants. None of them has been shown to be effective in treating infertility. The effectiveness of the other drugs described in this chapter has not been widely tested in clinical trials.

Recurrences of the disease are common following treatment with any of these drugs. About half the women using them will have a recurrence within a year.

Hormonal treatment is not an effective treatment for endometrial nodules, endometriomas or adhesions. If you wish to treat any of these you should have surgery rather than hormonal treatment.

Although all the hormonal drugs work in most cases, it is impossible to predict which drugs will work for you and whether the side effects will be tolerable. Hormonal treatment may be a process of trial and error before you find the one that suits you.

In addition, some of the drugs tend to be used in particular situations more commonly than others. For example, danazol, Synarel and Zoladex are frequently used as a first treatment to eradicate newly diagnosed endometriosis, or endometriosis that has recurred after some time. In contrast, Provera and the pill are more commonly used for women with chronic endometriosis to maintain suppression of symptoms following surgery or treatment with another drug. You may use different drugs as your situation changes.

About six to eight weeks after starting any course of treatment you should visit your gynaecologist to discuss how the treatment is progressing. Contact your gynaecologist if you develop any problems between scheduled visits.

The pill

The oral contraceptive pill is not just one drug. Rather, there are many different types of the pill and only some of them are used for treating endometriosis. Three of the more common brands used for endometriosis are Brevinor, Brevinor–1 and Norinyl–1.

The pill was first used to treat endometriosis in the late 1950s and for many years it was the preferred form of treatment. Today, it has been superseded by other drugs, so it is not normally used as a first treatment. Instead, it is more commonly used to achieve long-term suppression of the disease. That is, it is often used to stop the disease progressing in women with mild endometriosis or to stop the disease recurring following surgical or hormonal treatment.

How it works

When using the pill to suppress endometriosis, the aim of treatment is to reduce the number of periods as well as the amount of flow with each period. It is thought that this should lead to less retrograde menstrual fluid being deposited in the pelvic cavity, which in turn should reduce the likelihood of new implants developing.

Dosage

Many gynaecologists recommend the pill be taken every day for blocks of 3 to 4 months, followed by a break of a week during which you will have a light period. Taken in this way, treatment may continue for years.

Side effects

Some common side effects experienced when using the pill to suppress endometriosis include irregular vaginal bleeding, fluid retention, abdominal bloating, weight gain, increased appetite, nausea, headaches, breast tenderness and depression. Nausea and breast tenderness usually settle after 1 to 2 months of treatment. The remaining side effects usually disappear within a few weeks of finishing a course of treatment. Ovulation and normal menstrual periods usually resume within 4 to 6 weeks of finishing treatment.

Pregnancy and breastfeeding

There is no conclusive evidence to suggest that taking Brevinor, Brevinor–1 and Norinyl–1 during pregnancy will endanger the developing foetus, but it is probably best not to take the pill if there is any possibility you may be pregnant.

Small amounts of these three drugs have been found in the milk of breastfeeding mothers taking them and a few adverse effects on their infants have been reported. Therefore, these brands of the pill should not be used while breastfeeding.

Interactions

The pill interacts with some drugs so you should tell your gynaecologist if you are taking any other drugs.

Provera

Provera is commonly used to treat endometriosis. It is a strong progestogen (a synthetic progesterone-like drug) that is sometimes known by its chemical name medroxy-progesterone acetate and is sold under the brand names of Provera and Ralovera.

How it works

How Provera eradicates endometrial implants is not known precisely. It probably works by suppressing ovulation and inhibiting the growth of the endometrial implants, causing them to gradually waste away.

Dosage

Most gynaecologists recommend dosages of 30–60 milligrams a day for three to nine months. At these dosages, most women will stop ovulating and menstruating.

Although the usual length of short-term treatment is 3 to 9 months there is no evidence that prolonged or repeated courses of Provera cause long-term side effects.

Provera is sometimes used as long-term maintenance therapy for women with chronic endometriosis. In these cases, dosages of 30–60 milligrams a day are used initially to suppress the menstrual cycle and symptoms. The dosage is then gradually reduced to a level that just maintains suppression of symptoms. The dosage needed is usually 10–20 milligrams a day.

Side effects

For most women using Provera the side effects are mild to moderate in severity and are quite manageable. However, a few women will find them intolerable.

Many of the side effects are dose related—that is, the higher the dosage the more likely you are to experience side effects. Sometimes they can be controlled by reducing the dosage.

The more common side effects are spotting, irregular vaginal bleeding, depression, weight gain, bloating, fluid retention, headache, decreased libido, lethargy and tiredness, irritability, acne, nausea, breast tenderness and sweating.

The amount of weight gain on Provera varies widely. Most women will gain one or two kilograms but some women will experience larger gains.

You will usually begin to ovulate and menstruate again within 4 to 6 weeks of finishing treatment. The side effects are reversible and usually disappear within a few weeks of completing treatment.

Effectiveness

Little research has been carried out into the effectiveness of Provera for endometriosis. The results so far suggest that it is as effective as danazol in treating the pelvic pain associated with endometriosis, and that it does not improve the likelihood of pregnancy.

Pregnancy and breastfeeding

Provera should not be used during pregnancy as progestogens may cause abnormalities in the developing foetus. The use of Provera while breastfeeding is also not recommended. Small amounts of progestogens have been found in the milk of mothers taking them and the effect on the child is not known.

Interactions

There are no known interactions of Provera with any foods, alcohol or other drugs.

Depo-Provera

Depo-Provera is the long-acting injection form of Provera. It has been used to treat endometriosis for many years. It is also sold under the brand name of Depo-Ralovera and is sometimes known by its chemical name medroxy-progesterone acetate.

How it works

Depo-Provera is thought to eradicate endometrial implants in the same way as Provera.

Dosage

The dosages used vary. Some gynaecologists recommend one 50 milligram injection every week, or one 100 milligram injection every 2 weeks. Others recommend one 150 milligram injection every 2 to 3 months. The recommended length of treatment may vary from 6 months to a year or more.

Depo-Provera is a long-acting injection so any side effects experienced will persist until all the drug has been removed from your body. It has been suggested that women could try a short-term course of Provera tablets before embarking on a course of Depo-Provera injections. This would enable them to find out how their body responds to the drug and whether or not the side effects are likely to cause problems.

Side effects

The side effects of Depo-Provera include vaginal bleeding, weight gain, headaches, lethargy and tiredness, abdominal discomfort, dizziness, nervousness, decreased libido, back pain, leg cramps, depression, nausea, insomnia, acne, vaginitis, pelvic pain, breast tenderness, lack of hair growth, bloating, rash, fluid retention and hot flushes.

Vaginal bleeding is common and may be troublesome. The bleeding may be prolonged and heavy, or erratic with episodes of light bleeding or spotting.

Weight gain is also common and averages 2–3 kilograms after 12 months of treatment. The weight gain is usually greater with longer courses of treatment.

Most women will start ovulating and menstruating again within several months of their last injection. However, Depo-Provera sometimes causes a prolonged delay in the return of menstruation and a few women will not menstruate for more than a year following their last injection.

Therefore, this drug is not recommended for women who may wish to become pregnant soon after treatment.

Effectiveness

There is no reliable information on the effectiveness of Depo-Provera in treating endometriosis.

Pregnancy and breastfeeding

Depo-Provera has been used by a large number of pregnant women without causing any harmful effects in their unborn children. The use of Depo-Provera while breastfeeding is probably safe. No adverse effects have been detected in breastfed infants whose mothers were using Depo-Provera.

Interactions

There are no known interactions of Depo-Provera with any foods or alcohol but it does interact with the rarely used drug Cytadren (aminoglutethimide), which is used for Cushings syndrome and advanced breast cancer.

Duphaston

Duphaston has been used in Australia for over 30 years to treat women with endometriosis. It is sometimes also known by its chemical name dydrogesterone.

Duphaston is a progestogen (a synthetic progesterone-like drug) that is very similar to the naturally occurring progesterone produced by the ovaries.

How it works

It is not understood how Duphaston eradicates endometrial implants because, unlike the other drugs used to treat endometriosis, it does not stop menstruation nor does it usually stop ovulation at the dosages most commonly used.

It is thought that Duphaston probably works by inhibiting the growth of the endometrial implants in some way, causing them to gradually waste away.

Dosage

Most gynaecologists recommend 10–30 milligrams of Duphaston a day for 6 to 12 months. At these relatively low dosages, most women will continue to menstruate.

Side effects

Most women using Duphaston experience relatively few side effects. Those experienced are usually mild to moderate but they may be intolerable for some women.

The most common side effect is depression, which may be severe. Other side effects include nausea, breast tenderness, headaches, irregular bleeding, menstrual changes, fluid retention, weight gain and dizziness. The side effects of Duphaston are reversible and they disappear soon after treatment ceases. There are no known long-term side effects of Duphaston therapy.

Effectiveness

There is no reliable information on the effectiveness of Duphaston in treating endometriosis.

Pregnancy and breastfeeding

Duphaston should not be used during the first 4 months of pregnancy as it may cause abnormalities in the developing foetus. The use of Duphaston while breastfeeding is also not recommended. Small amounts of progestogens have been found in the breastmilk of mothers taking them and the effect on the child is not known.

Interactions

There are no known interactions of Duphaston with any foods, alcohol or other drugs.

danazol

Danazol has been used to treat endometriosis in Australia since the late 1970s. In the 1980s and early 1990s it was the most commonly used drug, but its use has declined in recent years. It is sold in Australia under the trade names of Danocrine and Azol.

Danazol is a weakened form of the male hormone testosterone. Testosterone is one of a group of male hormones known as the androgens that are produced by the male testes. They are responsible for the functioning of the male reproductive system and the development of the male characteristics such as facial hair and a deep voice. Androgens are also produced by the ovaries in very small amounts.

How it works

It is thought that danazol eradicates endometrial implants by several mechanisms. The net result is that oestrogen production is suppressed and the levels of oestrogen in the body decrease to the low levels found in women following the menopause. The low oestrogen levels mean the endometrial implants are no longer stimulated to grow and break down each month. Therefore, they become inactive and slowly degenerate.

Most women will stop ovulating and menstruating by the end of the second month of treatment, though this may depend on the dosage. The symptoms of endometriosis usually begin to diminish by the end of the second month.

Dosage

Most gynaecologists recommend that you begin with a dosage of 800 milligrams a day. Some research studies have suggested that danazol can be effective at lower dosages if your periods are suppressed. Once your periods have stopped, your gynaecologist may decrease your dosage to 600 milligrams or even 400 milligrams a day. The usual length of a course of treatment is 3 to 6 months but it may be extended to 9 months.

You should start your course of danazol on the first day of your period to decrease the risk of taking the drug during pregnancy. Although it is unlikely that you will conceive while on danazol, care should be taken to avoid pregnancy. It is recommended that barrier contraception (for example, condom or diaphragm or both) be used while taking the drug.

Side effects

Danazol can cause a wide variety of side effects and there is a huge variation in the way women respond to it. Most women experience some side effects and a few experience many. For some women the side effects are quite mild, but for others the side effects are severe and they are unable to complete a course of treatment.

The number and severity of side effects experienced is sometimes related to the dosage being taken. Reducing your dose to the lowest level needed to stop your periods may reduce the side effects experienced.

Some of the side effects of danazol are due to the fact that it is a weak synthetic male hormone. It may cause both androgenic (male characteristics) side effects and anabolic (body-building) side effects. The more common androgenic and anabolic side effects are acne, weight gain, fluid retention, deepening of the voice, increase in facial and body hair, oily skin and hair, change in appetite, bloating, decreased breast size, increased muscle bulk and enlargement of the clitoris.

Weight gain is by far the most common side effect. The majority of women experience weight gain—usually 1–5 kilograms but occasionally more. When treatment has finished most women lose much of the weight gain within 1 to 2 months but some find it difficult to lose the last kilogram or two.

Some women experience a change in their voice. The change may involve a loss of higher notes, or it may become husky, or it may peter out at times. If you notice any change notify your gynaecologist immediately as such changes may be irreversible.

Some women grow more facial hair. However, the facial hair is not usually noticeable to other people as it is only slightly more than normal and very fine and downy. If the hair growth is profuse notify your gynaecologist as this side effect is sometimes irreversible.

Enlargement of the clitoris is rare. However, if you notice any enlargement contact your gynaecologist immediately as it may be irreversible.

Some of the side effects of danazol are a result of the low levels of oestrogen in the body. These side effects are the symptoms usually associated with the menopause: hot flushes, night sweats and vaginal dryness.

Danazol can also cause a wide range of other side effects, including irregular vaginal bleeding or spotting, skin rash, nausea, vomiting, muscle cramps, joint soreness, joint swelling, headache, irritability, mood swings, anxiety, changes in libido, depression, hair loss, fatigue, liver disease, jaundice, increased cholesterol levels, decreased glucose tolerance and dizziness.

When you stop taking danazol you will usually start ovulating and menstruating within 4 to 6 weeks. Most of the side effects will disappear soon after completing treatment.

There is limited experience of long-term danazol therapy. However, toxicity and other problems of the liver have been reported.

Effectiveness

Danazol appears to be as effective as Dimetriose and the GnRH agonists (Synarel and Zoladex) in alleviating the symptoms of endometriosis, particularly in the early stages of the disease. Up to 80 per cent of women have had their symptoms of dysmenorrhoea, dyspareunia or chronic pelvic pain resolved or improved with danazol treatment. However, it does not increase the chance of pregnancy following treatment.

Pregnancy and breastfeeding

Danazol should not be used during pregnancy as it can cause masculinisation of the external genitals of a female foetus. If you suspect that you may be pregnant while taking danazol you should stop taking it and contact your gynaecologist immediately.

It is not known if danazol is excreted in the breastmilk nor whether it has any harmful effects on the infant, so it should not be taken while breastfeeding.

Interactions

There are no known interactions of danazol with any foods or alcohol. It can interact with some drugs so make sure that your gynaecologist is aware of any other drugs you are taking.

Dimetriose

Dimetriose is a relatively new drug that has been used to treat endometriosis in Australia since 1996. It is a synthetic hormone that is also known by its chemical name gestrinone.

How it works

Dimetriose eradicates endometriosis by several complex mechanisms. The net result of these mechanisms is that the endometrial implants are no longer able to grow and break down each month. Therefore, they become inactive and waste away.

Dosage

The usual dosage of Dimetriose is one 2.5 milligram capsule twice a week for 6 months. The first capsule should be taken on the first day of a menstrual period and the second capsule 3 days later. Thereafter, the capsules should be taken on the same days of the week every week and preferably at the same time of the day each time.

Occasionally, the gynaecologist will recommend that your dosage be increased to three capsules per week for a few weeks or for the remainder of treatment. This involves taking three capsules spread as evenly as possible over the week.

It is important to start your course of treatment on the first day of a period to minimise the risk of taking Dimetriose when you are pregnant.

It is recommended that you use non-hormonal forms of contraception throughout treatment (for example, condom or diaphragm or both). Dimetriose does not always stop ovulation and if you were to conceive it could cause abnormalities in the developing foetus.

Only one course of Dimetriose is subsidised under the Pharmaceutical Benefits Scheme—the scheme by which the Australian Government subsidises the cost of prescription drugs. The Government will subsidise only one six-month course of Dimetriose for each woman because of safety concerns about prolonged use.

Side effects

A large number of side effects have been reported with Dimetriose. Most women experience some of these side effects and a few experience many.

The more common side effects include weight gain, tiredness, acne, nausea, headaches, hunger, increased body hair, sweating problems, hot flushes, loss of libido, dizziness, leg cramps, swelling of the ankles and feet, skin rash, loss of appetite, voice changes, faintness, vomiting, depression and irritability.

The side effects usually disappear within a few weeks of finishing treatment but the weight gain may take longer to reverse. There is no information available on the long-term effects of Dimetriose.

Effectiveness

Dimetriose is as effective as danazol and the GnRH agonists (Synarel and Zoladex) in relieving symptoms and eradicating implants. It completely or partially relieves symptoms in about 80 per cent of women. Dimetriose has no effect on improving pregnancy rates.

Pregnancy and breastfeeding

Dimetriose should not be used during pregnancy as it has caused masculinisation of the external genitals of female foetuses in animal tests. If you suspect you may be pregnant you should stop taking the drug and contact your gynaecologist immediately.

It is not known if Dimetriose is excreted in breastmilk. However, a very similar compound known as norgesterol is passed into breastmilk so it is assumed that Dimetriose does likewise. Therefore, Dimetriose should not be taken while breastfeeding because it is likely to have harmful effects on the infant.

Interactions

There are no known interactions of Dimetriose with any foods or alcohol. However, the drug may not work properly if taken with some anti-epileptic drugs or with the tuberculosis drug, rifampicin.

Synarel and Zoladex

Synarel and Zoladex are two drugs from a group of drugs known as the GnRH agonists. They have been used to treat endometriosis in Australia since 1994.

Synarel, sometimes known by its chemical name naferelin acetate, comes in the form of a nasal spray. Zoladex, also known by its chemical name goserelin acetate, comes in the form of a monthly injection.

Synarel and Zoladex are modified versions of a naturally occurring hormone, gonadotropin releasing hormone, which helps to control the menstrual cycle.

How they work

Although Synarel and Zoladex come in different forms they work in exactly the same way. When used continuously for periods of longer than two weeks, Synarel and Zoladex stop the production of oestrogen by the ovaries through a series of mechanisms. They deprive the endometrial implants of oestrogen, causing them to become inactive and slowly degenerate.

Some women will experience 3 to 5 days of vaginal bleeding or spotting about 10 to 14 days after beginning treatment. Most women will stop bleeding within 2 months of starting treatment.

You should notice an improvement in your symptoms within 4 to 8 weeks of beginning treatment, but some women will experience a temporary worsening of symptoms in the first 2 weeks.

Dosage

The usual length of treatment with Synarel or Zoladex is 3 to 6 months. However, the actual dosage and mode of administration varies according to the drug being used.

One spray pump of Synarel contains enough Synarel to last 30 days of treatment. The recommended dosage is one spray of the pump into one nostril in the morning and one spray into the other nostril in the evening every day for 6 months. In a few women the recommended dosage does not stop menstruation. If symptoms persist in these women the dosage may be increased to one spray in both nostrils morning and night.

Zoladex comes as a long-term injection. The drug is embedded in a small biodegradable implant about the size of a grain of rice. The implant is injected just under the skin in the lower half of the abdomen. Once injected the implant slowly dissolves and releases the drug into the bloodstream over a period of at least 28 days. A course of treatment requires 6 consecutive injections each given 28 days apart.

You should not begin treatment if there is any possibility that you may be pregnant. Treatment with Synarel or Zoladex should begin on the first 2 to 4 days of your period to minimise the likelihood of starting the drug when you are pregnant.

Under most circumstances you are not likely to become pregnant while using Synarel or Zoladex. However, because of the possibility that these drugs may cause miscarriage or abnormalities in the developing foetus it is recommended that you use non-hormonal forms of contraception during treatment (for example, condom or diaphragm or both).

Only one 6-month course of either Synarel or Zoladex is subsidised under the Pharmaceutical Benefits Scheme. Because of the risks associated with repeated or prolonged use of Synarel and Zoladex, the Government will subsidise only 6 months of treatment for each woman.

Synarel and Zoladex often alleviate symptoms within 3 months. In these cases, many gynaecologists suggest that you only have 3 months of treatment initially so that you can save the remaining 3 months of your 6-month course for treatment at a later date if needed.

Side effects

The side effects of Synarel and Zoladex are a result of the low levels of oestrogen in the body. They are usually restricted to the symptoms associated with the menopause. The side effects are common and the overwhelming majority of women will experience at least one or two. The severity varies from mild to severe and unfortunately some women will find them intolerable.

Most women will experience hot flushes, or night sweats, or both. The other common side effects are decreased libido, headaches, mood swings, vaginal dryness, decreased breast size, increased breast size, acne, muscle pains and depression. These symptoms usually disappear soon after treatment ceases.

A small number of women will experience irritation of the nose from the spray when using Synarel, and some women will experience bruising and skin irritation at the site of the injection with Zoladex.

The return of ovulation and menstruation is variable. Most women will menstruate within 4 to 6 weeks of their last spray of Synarel or within 6 to 10 weeks of their last injection of Zoladex.

The most serious concern associated with the use of Synarel and Zoladex is the fact that both drugs cause a decrease in the density of the bones, particularly the bones of the spine. This decrease in bone density is in the order of 2.5–10 per cent at the end of a single 6-month course of treatment. There is evidence that much of the bone lost regenerates within six months of completing treatment and that 18–24 months after completing treatment probably most, if not all, of the bone lost is replaced.

A single 6-month course of treatment will not usually be detrimental for women with normal bone density. However, in women at risk for developing osteoporosis, treatment with Synarel or Zoladex could predispose them to developing the condition.

The single most important risk factor for osteoporosis is a history of the disease in a close relative, such as a grandmother or mother. If it is felt that you may be at risk of developing osteoporosis, you should consider having a bone density scan before embarking on treatment.

The menopausal and bone-loss side effects of treatment with Synarel and Zoladex can often be reduced by the use of add-back therapy. Add-back therapy involves taking just enough oestrogen to minimise the side effects while still allowing the drug to work effectively.

Effectiveness

Because Synarel and Zoladex destroy endometrial implants in the same way, they are equally effective in treating endometriosis. Both drugs are as effective as danazol in relieving symptoms and eradicating implants. They completely relieve or reduce symptoms in about 80 per cent of women. They have no effect on improving fertility.

Pregnancy and breastfeeding

Synarel and Zoladex should not be used during pregnancy as they may cause miscarriage or abnormalities in the developing foetus. It is not known if Synarel and Zoladex are excreted in breastmilk or if they have any harmful effects on the infant. Therefore, they should not be used while breastfeeding.

Interactions

There are no known interactions of Synarel and Zoladex with any foods, alcohol or drugs.

6
Surgical treatments

The main forms of surgery used to treat endometriosis are laparoscopy, laparotomy and hysterectomy. This chapter discusses each of these operations in detail.

Endometrial nodules, endometriomas and adhesions can only be treated surgically because hormonal treatments have no long-term effect on them. In addition, surgery may be necessary to correct any damage caused by the endometriosis.

Laparoscopy

A laparoscopy is an operation in which an instrument known as a laparoscope is used to diagnose and treat a range of gynaecological conditions, including endometriosis.

A laparoscope is a thin, telescope-like instrument approximately 30 centimetres long that is inserted into the pelvic cavity through a small cut near the navel. The instrument has a lens at the end that magnifies and lights up the pelvic cavity so the gynaecologist can see the organs and any endometriosis present. The laparoscope usually has a second tube attached along its length that is used to hold a variety of surgical instruments so the gynaecologist can perform surgical procedures during the laparoscopy. The operation generally takes from 30 minutes to two hours or more, depending on the severity of the endometriosis and what surgical procedures are done.

Originally, laparoscopy was used only as a means of diagnosing endometriosis but over the years it has been used increasingly as a way of surgically treating the condition.

Most gynaecologists are able to surgically treat endometriosis at the time of diagnosis and experienced surgeons are able to do complex procedures and treat more severe cases. The complexity of the procedures that your gynaecologist will attempt will depend on his or her level of training and experience, and the facilities available at the hospital where you are being treated.

Diagnostic laparoscopy

A diagnostic laparoscopy is one that is used only to diagnose endometriosis—no surgical treatment is attempted.

Operative laparoscopy

An operative laparoscopy is one in which various surgical procedures are carried out in order to treat any endometriosis and adhesions present. It can be performed at the time of diagnosis, which avoids the need to undergo a second laparoscopy to treat the endometriosis or to undergo hormonal treatment.

Preparation

Before your laparoscopy you should discuss with your gynaecologist what he or she proposes to do during your operation. If you have any procedures that you do or do not want done you should say so. If you are not sure that you have endometriosis you should discuss whether or not the gynaecologist intends treating the disease if it is found. Do not forget that because each case of endometriosis is different the gynaecologist will not know exactly what needs to be done until he or she has inspected your pelvic cavity. If you have any questions, make sure that you discuss them with the gynaecologist. If necessary, make a special visit to discuss the operation and resolve all your questions.

Before your laparoscopy, arrange for someone to be at home with you for the first day or so after the operation so they can look after you and help with household chores and child minding if necessary. If you have paid work make sure that you organise to have enough time off work after your laparoscopy. Some women need only one week's leave but others need longer, so try to organise two weeks off in case you need it—you can always return earlier if you are feeling well.

Operation

Hospital routines and practices vary. The information in this section is only a guide to what is likely to happen when you have your laparoscopy.

You should not have anything to eat or drink for at least six hours before the operation. If there is any possibility that you may have bowel surgery you will be given a solution to drink the day before your operation. The solution will clean out your bowel so that surgery can be done safely.

You will be admitted to the hospital a short time before your surgery is scheduled. The nurses will ask you questions about your general health, any medications you may be taking, and any previous operations you may have had. They will also take your blood pressure and pulse, possibly give you a pubic shave and give you a surgical gown to wear. The anaesthetist will visit you and ask questions about any allergies and problems you have had with previous operations.

When you go into the operating theatre, a general anaesthetic will be injected into a vein in your arm. A tube will be placed in your throat and connected to a machine that breathes for you.

You will be given a pelvic examination, and a hysteroscopy or D&C may be performed. A hysteroscopy is a procedure where a telescope-like instrument is inserted into the uterus through the vagina and cervix. It enables the gynaecologist to examine the inside of the uterus. A D&C, or dilation and curettage, is a procedure in which the cervix is dilated and the lining of the uterus is scraped with a spoon-like instrument known as a curette.

A small cut of about two centimetres will be made in or near your navel. Carbon dioxide gas will be pumped into your abdomen through the cut. The gas causes the organs in the abdomen and pelvis to separate from each other so the laparoscope can be safely passed into the pelvic cavity. The laparoscope is then inserted through the cut. The gynaecologist will make another small cut in the lower part of the abdomen so that an instrument can be inserted. The instrument is used to move the internal organs around so the gynaecologist can thoroughly inspect the entire pelvic cavity. Another instrument will be inserted into the opening of the cervix so the uterus can be moved back and forth as needed during the operation.

The gynaecologist will then carry out a thorough inspection of the pelvic cavity for signs of endometriosis. The instruments inserted through the lower cut and the cervix will be used to lift and move the uterus and ovaries around so their undersurfaces can be clearly seen.

The gynaecologist will be looking for endometrial implants on the ovary and the peritoneum overlying the pelvic organs. Black implants will generally be relatively easy to see but clear and red implants may be difficult to detect. Endometrial nodules are usually more difficult to see because they often lie below the surface of the peritoneum or only the tip of the nodule is visible. When looking for nodules the gynaecologist looks for any visible tips as well as bulges in the peritoneum that suggest a nodule may be underneath. Endometriomas may be seen lying on the surface of the ovary or the ovary may be enlarged, suggesting that an endometrioma lies within it. However, sometimes smaller endometriomas cannot be seen if they are embedded in the ovary. Adhesions will generally be obvious because of their characteristic appearance.

Once a diagnosis has been made the gynaecologist will mark the location of your implants, nodules, endometriomas and adhesions on a drawing or prepared chart. Because of the sometimes progessive and recurrent nature of endometriosis, it is important that an accurate chart of your endometriosis be made at the time of the laparoscopy. The chart will provide a record of the severity and extent of your endometriosis that can be compared with charts made during subsequent laparoscopies. This can give you and your gynaecologist a guide to the progression of your endometriosis and the effect of any treatments. If your gynaecologist does not give you a copy of the drawing or chart you may like to request one.

If you are having any operative procedures, the gynaecologist will make another two or three small cuts at various points in the lower abdomen. These cuts will be used to insert instruments for the surgical procedures, to remove samples of tissue, and to drain fluid from any endometriomas. The gynaecologist will then carry out any necessary surgical procedures, which are described in the following pages.

If fertility problems are present, dye may be passed through the fallopian tubes to see whether they are blocked.

When the operation has been completed and the details recorded, the laparoscope and other instruments will be removed and the carbon dioxide gas allowed to escape. The cuts will be protected with sticky plaster or tiny stitches and you will be taken to the recovery room.

Procedures

The procedures that may be performed as part of an operative laparoscopy include:

- removal or destruction of endometrial implants
- removal of endometrial nodules

- removal of endometriomas
- cutting of adhesions
- removal of ovaries
- surgery of the bowel or bladder
- presacral neurectomy or uterosacral neurectomy
- surgery to correct any other disease or abnormalities found.

Removal or destruction of implants

Endometrial implants are generally treated by one of two techniques: diathermy or excision. While every attempt is made to remove all the visible implants there are times when some implants must be left because the gynaecologist is not able to remove them without the risk of damaging underlying organs such as the bowel or ureter.

Diathermy involves destroying the implant by burning it with a heat gun or laser beam. Care must be taken when using the technique to ensure that only the implant is burnt and not any underlying tissue such as the bowel, bladder or ureter. The possibility of accidentally destroying underlying tissue means that most gynaecologists are wary of using diathermy on implants that lie on vital organs such as the bowel and large blood vessels. Care must also be taken to ensure that the entire implant is burnt so that it cannot regrow.

The excision of endometrial implants involves cutting out the implant so that a ring of normal tissue surrounds it when it is removed. The advantage of excision is that it allows the gynaecologist to separate the implant from the underlying tissue and ensure that the entire implant has been removed. Excision is a very useful technique to use when implants lie over vital organs such as the bowel and bladder because there is less risk of damaging the underlying organs. It also does not damage the implant so the gynaecologist is able to send a sample, known as a biopsy, to the pathologist to confirm that it is endometriosis.

Excision may be achieved with the use of scissors, a very fine heat gun, or a laser beam. Excision needs more skill and is more time consuming than diathermy, so it is not used by all gynaecologists.

Removal of nodules

Endometrial nodules are generally removed by excision so the gynaecologist can be sure that he or she has removed the entire nodule. If a nodule is large, the gynaecologist may have to dissect a considerable amount of tissue in order to excise it completely. The excision of nodules is generally achieved with the use of scissors or a laser beam. Removing nodules is technically very difficult and only a few gynaecologists are currently performing the procedure. The difficulty is due to the fact that most endometrial nodules lie in or near the Pouch of Douglas, the uterosacral ligaments and the rectovaginal septum. These areas lie close to the bowel and ureters and are easily damaged.

Removal of endometriomas

Endometriomas are usually removed by excising them. The endometrioma is first punctured and drained so the gynaecologist can see the fibrous wall that surrounds it. The wall is then stripped away from the surrounding ovary to ensure that the endometrioma is completely removed. Sometimes endometriomas are only drained, which often results in the endometrioma regrowing.

Cutting of adhesions

Adhesions that are not causing problems are best left alone but adhesions that are pulling and distorting organs or causing pain should generally be cut. The aim of cutting adhesions is to allow the organs to resume their normal position within the pelvic cavity. Adhesions can be cut with scissors, diathermy, or a laser beam. When cutting adhesions there is always a significant risk that the newly cut edges will again form adhesions. This tendency to form and reform adhesions is much greater in some women than in others and may be such a problem that further surgery to cut adhesions is not recommended. Sometimes the gynaecologist will wrap susceptible areas in a special cloth-like material known as Interceed to minimise the likelihood of adhesions developing between them. The material is absorbed by the body over the next 10 to 14 days, by which time the underlying tissues have had time to heal.

Removal of ovaries

Sometimes an ovary has to be removed because it is so severely diseased with endometriosis that it cannot be treated adequately or because an endometrioma lying within it cannot be removed safely. Sometimes, an adjacent fallopian tube must also be removed if it has been damaged.

Surgery of bowel or bladder

If endometrial nodules have penetrated the wall of the bowel, bladder or ureter and are causing problems, they must be removed carefully and the affected area repaired. Rarely, a section of the bowel will have to be removed if it has been severely damaged by endometriosis or adhesions.

Presacral or uterosacral neurectomy

Presacral neurectomy and uterosacral neurectomy are two procedures that are performed only occasionally in Australia, although they are performed more commonly overseas. Both involve cutting the nerves that transmit pain from the uterus to the brain in order to relieve chronic pain. At present there is no conclusive evidence that they are effective although there is some evidence that the procedures can cause side effects such as constipation.

Other surgery

If you have any other disease or abnormality of the organs in the pelvic cavity, these may be repaired by the gynaecologist.

Recovery

Immediately after the operation you will feel drowsy and have some abdominal pain. If you experience nausea or vomiting, the nursing staff can give you an injection to relieve it. You may have an intravenous drip in your arm to supply you with fluids.

When you are awake enough to comprehend and remember what is being said, your gynaecologist will come and discuss the results of your laparoscopy with you. He or she will explain the severity and location of your endometriosis as well as the nature of any surgical treatment that was done. Sometimes, the gynaecologist will leave you photographs of your operation or a diagram that shows the location of your endometriosis.

In most cases you will go home the same day. However, if you have severe pain or vomiting, you may need to stay in hospital another day or two.

For the first 1 to 2 days after your laparoscopy you will probably have generalised abdominal discomfort or pain. You may also experience abdominal bloating and mild to severe pain in the chest or shoulder region due to leftover carbon dioxide gas collecting under the diaphragm. Also, the tube that was placed in your throat may leave you with a sore throat for the first day or so. Over-the-counter painkilling tablets will usually be sufficient to relieve your pain.

Your cuts will probably have sticky plaster over them that will peel off after a few days. You may notice a little bruising around your cuts after a day or two. If a hysteroscopy or D&C was performed, you may have some bleeding or a discharge from the vagina.

Although a laparoscopy is said to be a minor operation, many women feel terrible afterwards. Many women say they feel like 'they have had ten rounds in the boxing ring' or 'have been run over by a truck!'

In most cases you will need a day or two in bed after the operation, preferably with someone around to keep an eye on you. It usually takes about five days before the symptoms of the operation subside. Most women take 5 to 7 days before they feel normal, although some will take up to two weeks to recover. Take your recuperation slowly and give yourself enough time to get over the operation.

You will usually be able to return to work sometime in the second week after the laparoscopy. Avoid strenuous exercise and lifting heavy weights for 1 to 2 weeks. Sexual intercourse and tampons should be avoided until any vaginal bleeding has stopped. Be guided by how you feel and do as much as is comfortable at the time.

You should notify your gynaecologist immediately if you develop any of the following symptoms:

- fever
- wound becomes painful, swollen and red
- discharge appears from wound
- severe abdominal pain or cramps
- frequent urination and scalding when passing urine
- vaginal discharge develops an unpleasant odour
- vomiting develops more than 24 hours after the operation
- tenderness and/or swelling in calf muscles
- increasing soreness of calf muscles when walking
- shortness of breath, chest pain or pain when breathing.

You will need to visit your gynaecologist 4 to 6 weeks after your laparoscopy to discuss your recovery, what was found during your operation, and your future management.

Risks and complications

A laparoscopy is a relatively safe operation. Most of the complications are minor and they usually resolve fairly quickly.

The rare complications that may occur during surgery include uncontrolled bleeding; damage to organs such as the bowel, bladder and large blood vessels; and gas embolus (a gas bubble entering a blood vessel and lodging in the lung). Complications that may develop after the operation include difficulty emptying the bladder, wound infection, urinary infection, infection of the uterus and vaginal discharge.

Effectiveness

It is impossible to give reliable figures on the success rates of laparoscopy. The results of research investigating the issue have been varied and confusing due to a number of factors, including the number of different procedures that are performed during laparoscopic surgery and the different levels of skill and experience of the gynaecologists performing the surgery. Nevertheless, it seems that the majority of women experience total or partial relief from their pain but a significant number experience a recurrence of their symptoms within a few years.

Laparotomy

Although endometriosis is usually treated surgically by laparoscopy there are times when the surgeon needs better visibility and more room than is possible when using a laparoscope. In these situations the surgeon must make a large cut in the abdomen. Such an operation is known as a laparotomy.

A laparotomy may be needed if an extensive mat of adhesions has fixed or distorted the arrangement of the pelvic organs. In this situation using a laparoscope would involve a risk of puncturing vital organs because the surgeon cannot see the organs properly and does not know if they are in their normal position. Certain procedures that are difficult to do with a laparoscope may need a laparotomy. Bowel surgery, removal of ovaries, removal of large endometriomas, and removal of endometrial nodules in the Pouch of Douglas and rectovaginal septum may come under this category.

Preparation

Before your operation, make sure that you and your gynaecologist agree on the purpose and nature of your surgery. In particular, make sure you discuss what procedures are likely to be performed. Tell the gynaecologist if there are any procedures that you particularly do or do not want done. Remember, however, that because each case of endometriosis is unique, until your gynaecologist looks inside your pelvis it is impossible to be sure what procedures will be needed. You should also discuss any questions or concerns you may have. If necessary, make a special visit to discuss these issues.

Preparation for your surgery should involve preparing yourself physically for the operation and planning for your recuperation. Generally, the healthier you are before surgery, the more quickly you will recover afterwards. It may be worthwhile taking a few steps to improve your general health before the operation. Measures worth considering include eating a nutritious diet, taking vitamin and mineral supplements, and exercising regularly. If you are a smoker, try to stop smoking at least 1 to 2 days, and preferably a week or more, before the operation to reduce the likelihood of anaesthetic complications. If you are taking the oral contraceptive pill, discuss with your doctor whether you should stop taking it before your surgery.

Before you go into hospital, arrange to have some help with household tasks such as child care, cooking, laundry and cleaning when you return home. If you have a job, arrange to have 6 to 8 weeks' leave so that you can fully recuperate before returning to work.

Operation

The practices and routines used by different hospitals vary. The information in this section should only be used as a guide to what may happen when you have your operation.

You should not have any food or drink for at least six hours before your surgery. If there is any possibility that you may need bowel surgery you will be given a solution to drink the day before that will clean out your bowel in readiness for the possible surgery.

You will usually go into hospital a couple of hours before your operation is scheduled. After being admitted to the ward the nursing staff will ask you questions about your health, any medications you may be taking, and any previous surgery you may have had. They will also prepare you for the operation by taking your blood pressure and pulse, shaving your pubic hair if necessary, and giving you a surgical gown to wear. The anaesthetist will visit you to discuss the operation and ask about any allergies and problems you may have had with previous operations. If you are apprehensive about your surgery, ask if you can have someone stay with you until you go into theatre.

Immediately before the operation you will be taken to the operating theatre. In the operating theatre a needle will be inserted into your arm and you will be given the general anaesthetic. After you have lost consciousness a tube will be placed in your throat and connected to a machine that breathes for you.

At the start of your operation the surgeon will make a cut about 10 centimetres long in your abdomen. This will usually be made along the pubic hairline. Sometimes the cut will be made vertically between the middle of the pubic hairline and the navel, particularly if you have had a vertical cut previously or if bowel surgery is likely. The gynaecologist will then thoroughly inspect the pelvic cavity for any signs of endometriosis, adhesions and other damage so that he or she can plan the operation and confirm what procedures need to be done. The procedures that are performed during a laparotomy are the same as those described for laparoscopy but they are done directly by the surgeon rather than with the aid of a laparoscope.

After the operation you will stay in the recovery room for half an hour to an hour before being taken back to your bed in the ward.

Recovery

After the operation you will have an intravenous drip in your arm to supply you with fluids because you will not be allowed to drink. You may have a catheter draining your bladder for the first day or two if you have had a hysterectomy. You may also have a tube coming out of the surgical wound to drain any excess fluid and debris from the area of the operation. Immediately after the operation you may have some nausea or vomiting. If this is troubling you, the nursing staff can give you an injection to relieve it.

You will usually feel drowsy and have some pain for the first few days after your surgery. The tube that was placed in your throat during the operation may give you a sore throat for the first day or so. Two to 4 days after your operation you will probably experience wind pain that can be uncomfortable.

For the first day or two you will be given painkilling drugs. You may have an analgesic pump so that you can give yourself pain relief when you need it, or you may be given the drugs continuously through your intravenous drip, or you may be given injections every 4 to 6 hours. You will then progress to tablets such as Panadeine Forte or Panadeine.

When you first start to drink again you will be allowed only to suck ice and sip small quantities of fluid. Once you are able to cope with fluids and any nausea and vomiting has ceased, your intravenous drip will be removed. You will then progress to a soft diet and later to a normal diet. You will probably not open your bowels for the first 2 to 4 days after your operation. If constipation becomes a problem you will be offered suppositories.

You will sit out of bed for a short time on the day after your operation and you will be encouraged to sit up and move around a little more each day as your condition improves.

You will probably be in hospital for 3 to 5 days. When you return home you will need another 3 to 5 weeks of recuperation if you have had a laparotomy; and another 3 to 7 weeks, and possibly up to 3 months, if you have had a hysterectomy. It is important that you move and walk around each day and gradually increase your activity level as you recover and feel better.

At first you will tire quickly so you will need help with cooking, laundry and cleaning for the first 1 to 3 weeks, particularly if you have children. When you start to do household jobs you should do only a little at a time and have plenty of rest in between. Do not try to be a superwoman as it will only slow down your recovery in the long term.

For the first week or two after you return home, you may still have some discomfort or pain so a mild painkiller such as Panadol or Panadeine may be necessary. If you have a vaginal discharge it will persist for about 2 weeks but it may last for 6 weeks or more following a hysterectomy.

It is advisable not to lift any heavy loads for about 6 weeks until your abdominal muscles have fully healed. You can drive a car again when you are confident that you can slam on the brakes without hurting your cut. You can have sexual intercourse again after you have visited the gynaecologist.

You should notify your gynaecologist immediately if you develop any of the following symptoms:

- fever
- cut becomes painful, swollen and red
- discharge appears from cut
- severe abdominal pain or cramps
- frequent urination and scalding when passing urine
- pain or bleeding when using bowels
- vaginal discharge develops an unpleasant odour
- vaginal discharge persists beyond 6 to 8 weeks
- tenderness and/or swelling in calf muscles
- increasing soreness of calf muscles when walking
- shortness of breath, chest pain or pain when breathing.

You should visit your gynaecologist about 6 weeks after your laparotomy to discuss your recovery, what was found during your operation, and your future management.

Risks and complications

A laparotomy is a relatively safe operation and the risks associated with it are fairly low. Most of the complications are relatively minor and resolve fairly quickly.

The rare complications that may occur during surgery include uncontrolled bleeding and accidental damage to internal organs, such as the bowel or bladder. Complications that may develop after the operation while you are still in hospital include paralysed bowel, bleeding at the wound site, urinary infection, wound infection, chest infection, heavy vaginal bleeding, difficulty emptying the bladder, thrombosis (when a blood clot forms in a vein, usually in the pelvis or a leg) and embolism (when a blood clot lodges in the lung).

Complications that may develop after you return home include wound infection, bleeding from the wound, urinary infection, vaginal discharge with an unpleasant odour and a change in bladder or bowel habits that may persist for 1 to 2 months.

Effectiveness

It is not possible to state the overall success rate of laparotomy. The figures vary widely and depend on which procedures were performed, the severity of the woman's endometriosis and the expertise of the gynaecologist performing the surgery, among other factors. It appears that laparotomy is beneficial in most cases but a significant number of women will have a return of their symptoms within a few years.

Hysterectomy

A hysterectomy for endometriosis is surgery that removes the uterus and as many remaining endometrial implants and adhesions as possible. One or both ovaries and fallopian tubes may also be removed.

A hysterectomy is usually performed only as a last resort to treat women whose endometriosis is so chronic and their symptoms so severe that their quality of life is intolerable. The most common reason that women with endometriosis have a hysterectomy is incapacitating pain. It should not be used—except in a few rare life-threatening situations—until a range of other treatments has been tried without success.

A hysterectomy is often said to be the only cure for endometriosis apart from the natural menopause. However, in a small proportion of women it does not cure the condition, especially if the ovaries are not removed.

Operation

There are two types of hysterectomy used for endometriosis. Sometimes only the uterus is removed. In this situation the woman will no longer menstruate but she will continue to ovulate until the time of her natural menopause. Sometimes the ovaries and fallopian tubes are removed as well as the uterus. In this situation, the woman will no longer menstruate or ovulate and she will undergo the menopause almost immediately.

A hysterectomy usually involves a laparotomy. All the details regarding laparotomy and its preparation and recovery apply to a hysterectomy, except that the procedures carried out also include removal of the uterus, cervix and possibly the ovaries and fallopian tubes as well. (See pages 79–85.)

In some circumstances, the gynaecologist may be able to perform a hysterectomy using a laparoscopy, or via the vagina, or using a combination of both methods. If you have a hysterectomy using any of these forms of surgery you will usually need to spend less time in hospital and have a shorter recuperation period. You should discuss with the gynaecologist whether one of these options is suitable for you.

Preparation

Whether or not to have a hysterectomy involves two or three separate decisions. First, you need to decide whether or not to have a hysterectomy. Second, whether or not to have your ovaries removed. Third, if your ovaries are removed, you need to decide if you are going to have hormone replacement therapy.

Hysterectomy or not?

When faced with the decision of whether or not to have a hysterectomy a woman has almost invariably had a harrowing and traumatic fight with unrelenting endometriosis for many years. Her symptoms are usually so severe and persistent that they have taken over her life and she has no other option. The decision to have a hysterectomy usually becomes a quality of life issue. Most women have to hit rock bottom and cross that 'invisible barrier' of knowing emotionally that they have reached the end of their tether before they can make the decision to have a hysterectomy.

Deciding to have a hysterectomy is a major and irreversible decision that will affect all aspects of your life. In making the decision you need to consider both the physical and emotional aspects.

You need to think about the degree to which your quality of life is being compromised by your endometriosis and weigh that up against the likely advantages and disadvantages the surgery will bring. Having a hysterectomy will probably mean much less pain and disability. It will also mean that you cannot have children in the future so you will have to decide if retaining your possible ability to have children is more important than relief from your symptoms and getting on with life. Your sexual response will probably change too—for better or worse—but you will not know how until after you have had the surgery.

You need to consider what effect not having all of your reproductive organs will have on your concept of yourself as a woman. Some women feel that removing their uterus means losing some of their 'womanhood' while others feel that their femininity has nothing to do with their uterus.

Make the decision at your own pace. Do not let yourself be pressured into making a hasty decision just because your gynaecologist or someone else wants an answer by a certain date. Only you will know when you have reached the end of your tether and have had enough, so take as much time as you need. If you have to ask yourself whether or not you are ready for a hysterectomy then you are probably not ready.

Also, the decision to have a hysterectomy should be yours and yours alone. Do not let anyone else—your gynaecologist, your partner, your mother, or your best friend—make the decision for you. You have to live with the decision, not them.

Before you make a final decision, get as much information as you need about the operation and its likely consequences. Do not hesitate to ask your gynaecologist any questions you may have. If you have any doubts about the need for the operation get a second, or even a third, opinion to make sure that you have exhausted all your options.

Discuss your options and your decision with your partner, family and friends, as well as other women who have been through the same operation. It may also be worthwhile talking to a counsellor if you are having difficulty resolving the issues. Remember, women who make the decision themselves and at their own pace usually recover more quickly and have fewer physical and emotional problems following their surgery.

Ovaries removed or retained?

The decision whether or not to have your ovaries removed is a complex and difficult one because there are no clear answers regarding the pros and cons of removing or retaining the ovaries. If your ovaries are removed you will no longer produce oestrogen, so you will undergo a premature menopause almost immediately—often within 24–48 hours. However, there will be less risk of your endometriosis recurring because the disease usually does not recur in the absence of oestrogen.

The symptoms of surgical menopause (menopause caused by surgical removal of the ovaries) are usually more severe than those experienced with the natural menopause. The drop in hormonal levels is both sudden and dramatic and many women will experience significant symptoms as a result. The most common early symptoms are hot flushes and night sweats. Some women will also experience tiredness and lethargy and sometimes depression if their hot flushes and night sweats interfere with their normal sleep. After a couple of months most women will start to experience some of the other effects of menopause. These include a dry vagina, a change in sexual response, decreased libido and decreased breast size. The main long-term effects of surgical menopause are an increased risk of developing heart disease and osteoporosis later in life.

If you retain your ovaries you will not undergo a premature menopause but there is a greater likelihood that your endometriosis will persist or recur because of the continued presence of oestrogen in your body. Unfortunately, it is not known how often endometriosis persists or recurs when the ovaries are retained.

There continues to be considerable debate among gynaecologists about whether the ovaries should be removed or retained. Some believe the ovaries should be removed because the risk of persistence or recurrence is too great if the ovaries are left and this risk outweighs the risks of premature menopause. Others believe that the ovaries should be retained because the risk of recurrence is low and the risks involved in a premature menopause are too great.

Although a number of gynaecologists routinely favour one option or the other, most base their recommendation on their assessment of the individual woman's needs. Therefore, you should find out what your gynaecologist intends to do and discuss your preferences. When you have made your decision, it is extremely important that you tell the gynaecologist whether you want your ovaries removed or retained.

Hormone replacement therapy or not?

If your ovaries are removed, the decision whether or not to have hormone replacement therapy (HRT) is also a difficult one because there is much debate about the use of HRT after removal of the ovaries for endometriosis. HRT is the use of synthetic hormones to replace the hormones that were previously produced by the ovaries in order to prevent or minimise the effects of menopause.

HRT usually involves the use of both synthetic oestrogen and progesterone but sometimes only synthetic oestrogen is used. The main forms of administration are tablets, implants and patches. There is a variety of dosages that can be used depending on the severity of your symptoms. The most common side effects are weight gain, nausea and sore breasts.

Using HRT will prevent or reduce most of the symptoms of surgical menopause, including hot flushes, night sweats and a dry vagina. It will also reduce the likelihood of you developing heart disease or osteoporosis later in life. However, there is a risk that the oestrogen component will lead to a persistence or recurrence of any endometriosis left in your body. Nevertheless, many gynaecologists believe that, because the amount of oestrogen used is much smaller than that produced by the ovary, the risk of recurrence is very small.

Some gynaecologists recommend that you wait 3 to 6 months after your hysterectomy before starting HRT. This delay should allow any remaining endometrial implants to degenerate and waste away, thereby reducing the chances of a persistence or recurrence. Other gynaecologists suggest that using only a synthetic progesterone such as Provera, rather than both oestrogen and progesterone, as an interim measure for the first few months will reduce the likelihood of recurrence while still providing some relief from the early symptoms of surgical menopause.

If you are unlucky enough to have a recurrence of your symptoms of endometriosis while on HRT, it may be possible to treat the recurrence by reducing the dosage or stopping it altogether. It may also be possible to treat the endometriosis by having a course of a hormonal treatment such as Provera.

If you do not take HRT you will have less chance of having a persistence or recurrence of your endometriosis. However, you will probably experience the effects of surgical menopause and you will have an increased risk of developing heart disease and osteoporosis later in life.

If you choose not to take HRT you may be able to prevent or minimise the symptoms of surgical menopause by eating a good diet, particularly one rich in foods containing phyto-oestrogens (natural oestrogens) such as grains and soy products. Other measures include taking vitamin and mineral supplements, having regular vigorous exercise and regular sexual activity. Even if these measures are not successful some women find that the symptoms of surgical menopause are preferable to their endometriosis symptoms and therefore they choose not to take HRT for fear of stimulating their endometriosis again.

7
Self-help and complementary therapies

Chronic endometriosis is a complex disease that does not always respond to conventional western medicine. Consequently, many women have turned to self-help and complementary therapies to augment, or replace, conventional hormonal and surgical treatments.

There is a wide range of self-help and complementary therapies used to treat women with endometriosis, although very little research has been done on their effectiveness. One of the few studies that has investigated the issue was done by the North American-based Endometriosis Association. The study involved 4000 women with endometriosis who were asked what alternative treatments they had tried and whether or not the treatments had helped. The survey received 2293 responses to the question regarding alternative treatments and the results are shown in Table 7.1.

The results of the study suggest that a wide range of self-help and complementary therapies can benefit women with endometriosis. This chapter outlines the more common therapies used in Australia.

Self-help

Paying attention to lifestyle factors that influence your health will enhance your overall health and wellbeing. Being healthier will, in turn, improve your body's chances of coping with and perhaps overcoming your endometriosis. This section deals with four lifestyle factors that you can work on to improve your overall health and wellbeing.

Table 7.1 Did the alternative treatment help?

Treatment	Yes (%)	No (%)
Candidiasis	65	20
Exercise	63	20
Change in diet	62	21
Counselling	59	24
Acupuncture and acupressure	56	27
Vitamins and minerals	56	19
Traditional Chinese herbs	49	24
Other herbs	49	26
Aromatherapy	48	26
Immunotherapy	48	30
Chiropractic	47	34
Homeopathy	41	33

Note: Immunotherapy is rarely used in Australia so it has not been described here.

Exercise

Most people know about the importance of exercise in preventing heart disease, but few people understand the role of exercise in promoting wellbeing. Mild exercise promotes a sense of wellbeing, elevates mood, alleviates the symptoms of stress and depression, stimulates better digestion and enhances the removal of waste products. These benefits are not confined only to healthy people. Rather, they are of greater importance in people with chronic illness and pain. Inactivity contributes to the feelings of being unwell and miserable, and reduces the ability to deal with the stresses of daily life.

The benefits of exercise can be gained through as little as 20 to 30 minutes of gentle exercise three or four times a week. Suitable activities include walking, cycling and swimming. If you have not exercised recently, start with 5 to 10 minutes at a time and gradually build up the duration as your fitness and tolerance improve. If you have chronic pain, find a form of exercise and a time of day to exercise that minimises your pain.

Diet

Eating a healthy and well-balanced diet promotes general health and wellbeing. Improving your diet is a good way of giving your body the best chance of healing itself. Eating lots of fresh fruit, vegetables and whole grains will give you a diet that is high in fibre, minerals and vitamins, and low in fats, sugars and salts.

Nutrition is one of the foundations of naturopathy. Naturopaths can provide advice on diet, help you create a diet that is suited to your needs, and make recommendations about any nutritional deficiencies you may have. They can also advise you on how to stimulate the immune system through diet. Dieticians and GPs with an interest in nutrition can also provide this advice.

Rest and relaxation

Adequate rest and relaxation are essential for good health and optimum functioning of the immune system. Make sure that you get enough sleep each night and have at least 20 minutes of relaxation during the day. Your relaxation may involve having a bath, listening to some good music, reading a book, chatting with a friend, or going for a walk. If you are stressed or find it difficult to relax, try some of the relaxation techniques described in Chapter 8 (on pages 110–12) or obtain some relaxation tapes from your local library or bookshop.

Stress management

Stress is not a cause of endometriosis but it will reduce your ability to cope with the disease. If you can deal more effectively with the stressors in your life you will be able to cope better and you will probably find your symptoms less troublesome.

There are many aspects to stress management. The aspects you need to focus on will depend on your particular needs and weaknesses. Some of the skills and activities that have helped women manage stress better include exercising regularly, having relaxation time every day, developing better sleep habits, learning to be assertive, developing better communication skills, managing time better, learning to solve problems, improving self-esteem, and being motivated.

There are many courses and books available on stress management. Think about enrolling in a course or reading a book on an aspect of your life that is difficult. Developing better life habits and skills will enable you to manage the stress in your life more effectively.

Complementary therapies

This section covers a range of complementary therapies that have been used to treat women with endometriosis. Each description gives a brief outline of the main philosophy and practices of the therapy to help you choose the ones you might like to try. Some of the therapies can be self-administered but you are strongly advised to seek professional help or research the field thoroughly before doing so.

The results of the study by the Endometriosis Association suggest there is not a lot of difference in the success of the various therapies (see Table 7.1), so choose the therapies you want to try on the basis of what seems 'right' for you and then see how you respond to them. It is sensible to start with just one or two so that you can get a clearer idea of which ones are working. Like conventional western treatments, the process of finding the best combination will probably be a matter of trial and error.

Having chosen the therapies you want to try, you need to find a practitioner who will treat you and with whom you feel comfortable and confident. Every practitioner of complementary therapies has their own ideas about the best way to treat endometriosis and there is little consistency in the way different practitioners treat the condition. You may need to do your homework when choosing a practitioner. In particular, find out what therapies they use and their approach to treating endometriosis. You may like to refer to pages 146–8 in Chapter 12 for possible pointers to consider when choosing a practitioner.

You should also find out if your potential practitioner is qualified and registered by the relevant professional body to practise in their field. Their certificates will usually be displayed in their consulting rooms if they are qualified and registered. If not, do not hesitate to ask them about their qualifications.

Naturopathy

Naturopathy is a philosophy of healing that uses natural methods to prevent and cure disease. It is based on the belief that the body has an innate ability to heal itself given the right conditions. The current system of naturopathy developed during the eighteenth and nineteenth centuries but the origins can be traced back to about 400BC.

Naturopathy treats the whole person, including their emotional and spiritual states. Where possible, it focuses on the underlying causes of ill health rather than only treating the symptoms. The naturopath is also seen as being an adviser and teacher of how to maintain good health in the long term rather than just a healer.

Naturopathy uses a wide range of therapies, including herbal medicine, homeopathy, vitamins and minerals, nutrition, hydrotherapy, Bach flower remedies and reflexology. The therapies used will depend on a variety of factors, including the naturopath's expertise and your condition, circumstances and preferences.

Naturopathy is especially effective in the treatment of chronic candidiasis, a condition sometimes found in women with endometriosis. Chronic candidiasis is an excessive build-up in the levels of a yeast, *Candida albicans*, that occurs naturally in the body. This build-up causes a range of symptoms, including recurrent or persistent vaginal thrush, recurrent or chronic skin infections, tiredness and lethargy, insomnia, food cravings, food and chemical allergies and digestive symptoms. Some factors that contribute to the development of chronic candidiasis are antibiotics, immunosuppressive drugs such as cortisone, birth control pills and a high-carbohydrate diet.

Treatment of chronic candidiasis includes medication to reduce the levels of yeast in the body, creating a yeast-free diet and avoiding yeasts in the environment. Your naturopath will also work with you to identify any food and chemical allergies, and vitamin and mineral supplements that will help your body overcome the excessive levels of yeast.

Western herbal medicine

The ancient art of western herbal medicine uses plants to prevent and treat illness. The herbal preparations are derived from various parts of the plant and there are herbal remedies for just about every condition. The herbs are used to create the ideal environment for health and self-healing.

Each herbal remedy is prepared by the herbalist especially for the person being treated. The herbs may be taken in a variety of forms. They may be dried and used in a tea, or taken as a tablet. More commonly, they are extracted from the plant using water or alcohol to make a tincture or concentrated drops of the herb. Some herbs are quite safe and well known but others can be toxic and should only be taken in consultation with a herbalist.

Vitamins and minerals

A range of vitamin and mineral supplements can be used to enhance general health and overcome illness. Naturopaths or GPs with an interest in nutritional medicine are probably the best sources of guidance on using vitamin and mineral supplements.

Homeopathy

Homeopathy, which was first developed by Samuel Hahnemann in 1755, uses very small doses of specially formulated remedies to promote healing. There are thousands of potential remedies but there are no specific remedies for particular conditions. Instead, the remedy for a patient is specially selected to treat that person's combination of physical, mental and emotional symptoms. The remedies work by stimulating the person's immune system and powers of recovery, thereby allowing them to cure themselves.

Massage

Massage is a form of healing dating back to about 400BC. It has evolved separately in various parts of the world so there are now many different forms of massage, including shiatsu, reflexology and relaxation. Massage promotes mental wellbeing through relaxation and its physical effects include pain relief, improved blood flow and enhanced cleansing in some tissues.

Reflexology

Reflexology is a form of massage of the feet that dates back to ancient Egypt and China. It is based on the idea that energy flows through the body in channels that link the organs and tissues of the body to specific points in the foot known as reflex points.

The reflex points are used to diagnose disease. Pressure applied to an organ's reflex point causes discomfort at the reflex point if the organ is diseased. The points are also used to heal. Massaging an organ's reflex point for a few minutes until the pain eases stimulates the flow of energy to the affected organ which in turn promotes healing.

Aromatherapy

Aromatherapy uses the aromas of about 60 essential oils to enhance vitality and treat a range of ailments. The aromas have a stimulating and healing effect on the tissues and organs. The essential oils are derived from a variety of plants, including trees, bushes, herbs and flowers.

The oils can be applied in several ways: they can be rubbed into the body by massage, added to bath water, or used in a compress. The oil can also be vaporised in an oil burner so the room is filled with its scent.

Bach flower remedies

Bach flower remedies use the essences of certain flowers to transform people's negative emotions. The therapy was developed by Dr Bach, who believed that physical illness was a reflection of the person's mental attitude. He discovered that extracts of certain flowers could relieve emotional distress and allow the person to recover more quickly from physical illness. Thirty-eight remedies are used to treat apprehension, indecision, loneliness, insufficient interest in circumstances, over-sensitivity, despondency, despair and over-care for others.

Traditional Chinese medicine

Traditional Chinese medicine has been used in China for the last 4500 years. It is based on the belief that energy flows through the body along channels known as meridians, and that any blockage of this energy flow leads to problems and, eventually, disease.

Chinese medicine uses a variety of therapies, including Chinese herbal medicine, acupuncture, massage and exercise. Since lifestyle is seen to be an important factor in health, Chinese medicine also looks at the person's diet, work patterns and methods of dealing with stress. Chinese herbs are used to encourage the person's inherent ability to heal and cope with their condition. Each combination of herbs is precisely designed for the person's specific collection of symptoms. The person prepares their own herbal preparation by boiling the recommended herbs into a soup that is taken morning and night.

Acupuncture and acupressure

Acupuncture is a form of traditional Chinese medicine. Its purpose is to restore a more normal and balanced energy flow to the body. The energy flow is stimulated by inserting needles at specific points along the meridians known as acupuncture points.

Acupressure originated as a first-aid technique. It is based on the same principles as acupuncture but the acupuncture points are stimulated by finger pressure instead of needles. Acupressure is easy to learn and you can do it on yourself or have a friend do it for you.

Shiatsu

Shiatsu is a traditional Japanese method of healing based on the principles of Chinese acupuncture, but instead of needles the practitioner uses his or her body to massage the areas where the energy flow is blocked. The practitioner may use anything from finger and thumb pressure to elbow and knee pressure. The aim of treatment is to reinforce or re-establish the body's ability to function normally and to stimulate the immune system.

Meditation

Meditation is an ancient eastern technique that relaxes the mind and body by inducing a trance-like state. There are many different forms, including bubble (thought) meditation, mantra (word) meditation, and zazen (breath) meditation. The aim of meditation is to cut off all sensory input to the brain—the sights, sounds, smells and thoughts that go with everyday life—thereby giving the mind and body a chance to rest properly.

Yoga

Yoga is an oriental philosophy and practice that involves learning a range of postures, and breathing and relaxation exercises. It is commonly seen as a system of stretching and relaxation but it can also be used to relieve symptoms and treat a range of ailments. Ideally, when using yoga for therapeutic purposes, the exercises should be adapted for your particular needs or they could aggravate your condition. If possible, one-to-one instruction should be sought from a yoga instructor rather than just attending group classes.

Chiropractic

Chiropractic medicine focuses on the joints and muscles of the body, particularly those of the spine. It is based on the idea that the role of the spine is to protect the spinal cord and its associated nerves so it must be in perfect alignment. If the spine is out of alignment the nerves coming from the spinal cord at that point will become irritated. This leads to poor functioning and possibly disease in the organs and tissues connected to the nerve.

Chiropractic treatment involves manipulating the joints and muscles of the spine to restore perfect alignment and allow the body to heal itself. The manipulation may comprise gentle stretching and mobilisation of the joints, and massage of the back muscles. Treatment may be followed by exercises that maintain the alignment.

Counselling

Counselling helps people deal with the emotional problems that are restricting their lives. As such, counselling can help women come to terms with their feelings and reactions regarding their endometriosis and its impact so they can cope better. For example, counselling can help women deal with any anger, depression, and family or relationship problems that have resulted from their endometriosis. It can also help women come to terms with specific issues such as hysterectomy and infertility. Counsellors can also teach skills that will help women deal with any future problems more effectively.

8
Pain management

Pain is the dominant symptom for many women with endometriosis, but, unfortunately, there has been little research into the nature and treatment of endometriosis pain. As a result, not a lot is known about endometriosis pain and treatment is based on what has been successful for pain in general. This chapter looks at pain, the possible causes of endometriosis pain, and ways of managing both short-term and long-term pain.

Causes of endometriosis pain

Pain is a message that tells us a part of the body has been damaged in some way. The message is transmitted by a network of nerves from the site of the damage to the brain where it is perceived as pain. No-one knows exactly what causes the pain associated with endometriosis, but it is likely there are several causes.

It is thought that much of the pain of endometriosis, especially that experienced during menstruation, occurs when the younger implants bleed onto the surrounding peritoneum. This bleeding causes inflammation and the release of pain-producing chemicals known as prostaglandins, which in turn causes pain. It is also possible that bleeding into older implants and nodules causes pressure and hence pain in much the same way that a boil causes pain.

Stretching and pulling of adhesions can cause pain. Adhesions on the surface of the ovary may cause pain during ovulation and menstruation if they are stretched when the ovary swells slightly at those times. Adhesions on the bowel may cause pain because they are often stretched and pulled as the bowel moves around during normal digestion.

Although it is very rare, rupture of an endometrioma may also cause pain because the spillage of its contents severely irritates the surrounding tissues, causing inflammation and the release of pain-causing prostaglandins.

Using pain medications

Analgesics, more commonly known as painkillers, are designed to control short-term, mild to moderate pain. They are not designed to control chronic or long-term pain and their use is fraught with danger if they are taken inappropriately for long periods of time.

Using analgesics intermittently to control pain, such as for a few days each month to control period pain or ovulation pain, is quite acceptable. However, using analgesics for most of the month can, and often does, lead to reduced effectiveness of the drug and long-term problems for the woman. With prolonged, regular use, the body develops a tolerance to the analgesic being used. This means that larger and larger doses are needed to achieve the same effect. As a result, women find they need to take larger doses more frequently in order to control their pain. They also find that they need to use increasingly stronger analgesics to achieve the same level of control. Unfortunately, the stronger analgesics contain morphine-like drugs that can be highly addictive if used indiscriminately.

Types of pain medications

Analgesics are drugs that control pain by stopping the transmission of the pain message at some point along its pathway. There are several types: simple analgesics, compound analgesics, narcotic analgesics, non-steroidal anti-inflammatory drugs and antidepressant drugs. It must be

Table 8.1   Pain medications

Type	Brand names
Simple analgesics	
(i) Aspirin-based	Aspro, Dispirin and Solprin
(ii) Panadol-based	Dymadon, Panadol, Panamax, Paralagin and Tylenol
Compound analgesics	
(i) Milder	Aspalgin, Codalgin, Codiphen, Codis, Codral Pain Relief, Dymadon Co, Fiorinal, Mersyndol, Mersyndol Day Strength, Panadeine, Panadeine Plus, Panamax Co and Veganin
(ii) Stronger	Capadex, Codral Forte, Di-Gesic, Mersyndol Forte and Panadeine Forte
Narcotic analgesics	Endone, Fortral, Morphine, Percodan, Pethidine, Proladone
Non-steroidal anti-inflammatory drugs	ACT–3, Actiprofen, Brufen, Naprogesic, Naprosyn, Nurofen, Ponstan
Antidepressant drugs	Aropax, Efexor, Prothiaden, Prozac, Serzone, Sinequan, Tofranil, Tryptanol, Zoloft

remembered that pain medications treat only the pain of endometriosis—they have no effect on the disease itself.

Simple analgesics

The simple analgesics are aspirin and paracetamol. Both are highly effective in relieving mild to moderate pain. They can be purchased without a prescription from chemists and supermarkets.

The main side effects of aspirin are irritation and bleeding of the stomach. These effects can usually be avoided by taking the drug with food or a glass of milk. Paracetamol does not cause irritation or bleeding of the stomach.

Compound analgesics

The compound analgesics are a group of analgesics that contain a combination of either aspirin or paracetamol and a mild narcotic (morphine-like drug) such as codeine or dextropropoxyphene hydrochloride. The milder compound analgesics contain either aspirin or paracetamol and 8–10 milligrams of codeine. They are available without a prescription from pharmacies.

The stronger compound analgesics contain either aspirin or paracetamol and 30 milligrams of codeine or 32.5 milligrams of dextropropoxyphene hydrochloride. They are only available on a doctor's prescription. Codeine is a mild narcotic that can cause constipation at relatively small doses. It should be used with care or avoided if you have bowel symptoms that are exacerbated by constipation. Codeine is also addictive, especially if taken in large amounts or for prolonged periods. The stronger compound analgesics containing codeine should only be used for a few days at a time.

Narcotic analgesics

The narcotic analgesics are a group of strong analgesics that are similar to morphine. Because they are addictive, they should be used only under strict medical supervision and in limited quantities for severe short-term pain. Some of the better known narcotics include Endone, Fortral, Morphine, Percodan, Pethidine and Proladone.

The side effects of narcotic analgesics include nausea, constipation, drowsiness, slow breathing and mood changes. The other potential problems are tolerance and addiction. In rare cases where long-term narcotics are needed, the risk of addiction is less if longer-acting narcotics such as MS Contin are used. Nowadays, however, non-narcotic drugs such as Tramal are preferred because they are less addictive.

Non-steroidal anti-inflammatory drugs

The non-steroidal anti-inflammatory drugs are a group of drugs commonly used in the treatment of arthritis. They relieve inflammation and pain by blocking the production of pain-producing chemicals known as prostaglandins. These medications may be effective for dysmenorrhoea and other pain due to endometriosis provided that they are taken correctly.

Since the non-steroidal anti-inflammatory drugs work by blocking the production of pain-causing chemicals, they must be taken before any of these chemicals are produced. Therefore, you must start taking them at least 24 hours before you expect to experience pain. If you delay taking them until after you feel pain they cannot do anything about the pain-producing chemicals that have already been made so they will not alleviate your pain.

If you are using non-steroidal anti-inflammatory drugs for ovulation pain or period pain, start taking them at least 24 hours before you expect to ovulate or start bleeding. If you have an unpredictable menstrual cycle, you can safely take them for a week or more before you expect the pain. Once you have started taking them it is also important to take them regularly every six hours so that no pain-producing chemicals are made when you ovulate or your period starts.

Brufen and Naprosyn need a doctor's prescription but the other non-steroidal anti-inflammatories can be bought over the counter from chemists. Ponstan can also be bought in small quantities over the counter but larger quantities are available with a doctor's prescription.

Responses to the different brands vary. You may need to try more than one brand before you find one that relieves your pain. A bonus of taking some of the non-steroidal anti-inflammatories such as Ponstan and Naprogesic is that they decrease the amount of menstrual bleeding by up to a third.

The most common side effects of the non-steroidal anti-inflammatories are nausea, vomiting, diarrhoea, irritation of the stomach and stomach ulcers. These can usually be minimised if you take the tablets with food or a drink of milk.

Antidepressant drugs

Antidepressant drugs are sometimes used to treat chronic pain. They are taken to enhance the pain-relieving effects of analgesics by overcoming the depression that often develops as a result of chronic pain.

The more common antidepressants used to help manage pain include Aropax, Efexor, Prothiaden, Prozac, Serzone, Sinequan, Tofranil, Tryptanol and Zoloft. New types of anti-depressant drugs have been released in recent years and more will be released soon. If you are using antidepressants to help manage your chronic pain, talk to your GP to make sure that you are on the most appropriate medication for your needs.

Managing chronic pain

Using analgesics for prolonged periods can lead to tolerance and addiction. Therefore, if you have pain for much of the month you need to think about other ways of managing it.

Before you think about managing your long-term or chronic pain you need to make sure that nothing more can be done to treat the cause. If the pain is due to your endometriosis or adhesions, you need to be sure that you have exhausted all possible treatment options.

Managing chronic pain is a specialised field that needs a team of trained and experienced people. If you have chronic pain that is interfering with your daily life you need more specialised help than your GP can offer. You will probably need to seek help from a pain clinic—it could make the difference between having a life controlled by pain and leading a relatively normal life.

Although it will be difficult for you to accept, the current philosophy of managing chronic pain assumes that you will not be able to eliminate your pain all the time. In other words, you will have to learn to live with some pain at least part of the time. The aims of managing chronic pain are to achieve a reasonable level of pain control and to increase your coping skills and control over your life.

Analgesics are used continuously around the clock in a scheduled regime rather than just when you need them. The dosage used is the minimum needed to achieve a reasonable level of pain control most of the time—for example, you may take the prescribed dose every four hours. This regime minimises the risk of physical and psychological addiction while allowing you to have enough control to have a reasonable quality of life.

Having achieved a reasonable level of pain control, learning to manage chronic pain involves changing the way you think about your pain and its impact. Rather than focusing on your pain and the fact that you cannot eliminate it, you need to learn to focus on making the best of the times when you do have control and learning to ride the times when you do not have full control. Needless to say, this is difficult and requires help from trained specialists. However, it can be done and is well worth the effort.

To manage chronic pain successfully you also need to feel in control. You will need to spend time thinking about your life and its direction, improving your self-confidence, learning to think more positively, and learning new coping skills—all of which will help you to regain control. Pain clinics provide psychologists, physiotherapists, occupational therapists and other staff who can help you develop the necessary skills.

Other techniques to help manage pain

Analgesics may not completely alleviate your short-term or long-term pain, or there may be times when you do not want to use them. There is a range of techniques for managing pain that you may want to try. These techniques can be used on their own or in combination with analgesics.

Heat

You will probably have already discovered that heat brings relief from pain, especially period pain. The faithful hot water bottle placed on the affected area can diminish your pain significantly. Other forms of heat relief include wheat packs, electric blankets, heating pads, hot showers, baths and spas.

Exercise

Many endometriosis sufferers feel they cannot exercise because of chronic pain. However, exercise is important in controlling pain because it gives you a feeling of wellbeing and increases the production of endorphins, the natural painkilling chemicals produced by the body. For further information see pages 93–4 in Chapter 7.

Tai chi

Tai chi was developed in China many hundreds of years ago. It consists of a series of slow, dance-like movements. Using correct breathing, controlled stretching, and gentle artistic movements, tai chi is a graceful way of exercising without much effort.

Relaxation

Relaxation techniques are commonly used to help manage chronic pain. Many women with chronic pain forget how to relax. Relearning takes time and practice, but, once mastered, relaxation will reduce your pain and improve your overall wellbeing.

Pain is a vicious cycle. It causes fear, stress and anxiety, which leads to tensing of the muscles, which in turn further increases the pain. When you are tense and anxious you use more energy, which leaves you feeling drained and exhausted. If you can break the cycle of pain, tension, more pain and exhaustion by learning to relax at will, you will reduce your pain. There are several ways of learning to do this. Here are two techniques to try.

Controlled breathing

Controlled breathing is one of the oldest and simplest relaxation techniques. It can enable you to relax tense muscles, slow your heart rate and lower your blood pressure.

Find a place where you can be undisturbed for half an hour and where you can sit or lie in a well-supported and comfortable position. Close your eyes and try to relax your body. Now take deep, slow breaths in through your nose and out through your partly closed lips. Concentrate on the rhythm of breathing in and out and feel your tension begin to melt away. Try to maintain this slow, deep, rhythmic breathing for 15 minutes. The technique should be performed at least once a day to get maximum relief.

Progressive muscle relaxation

Progressive muscle relaxation can be helpful if your muscles are tense and tight as a consequence of your pain.

Find a comfortable place where you will be undisturbed for about 20 minutes. Start by taking slow, deep breaths. As you breathe, concentrate on curling up your toes and tightening them as hard as you can. Maintain this tension and tightness in your toes and feet for about 10 seconds and then relax them completely. You will notice how the toes uncurl and your feet become heavy. Feel the contrast between your tensed and relaxed muscles.

Gradually move your attention up your body, systematically tensing and relaxing the muscles of your legs, thighs, buttocks, abdomen, shoulders, arms, hands, neck, jaw and face. As you continue to work through this technique, take particular note of the contrast between tense and relaxed muscles. With practice you will be able to relax your muscles when they tighten in response to pain.

Imagery

Imagery, or visualisation as it is sometimes called, will not get rid of your pain. Rather, it will give you time out by allowing you to use your imagination to create mental images that block out the pain.

The aim of imagery is to fill your mind with positive images to replace the negative ones caused by your pain. For example, you may imagine that you are in an open paddock on a warm sunny day. Beside you is a helium-filled balloon with a large basket attached. You fill the basket with your pain. The balloon now rises up and floats away, taking your pain with it. Alternatively, you may imagine that your endometriosis is being invaded by an army of white blood cells. The white blood cells destroy the unwanted endometriosis cells and leave you with a healthy, pain-free body.

Positive thinking

Negative thoughts about pain cause stress, tension, anxiety and, ultimately, more pain. If you can replace your negative thoughts and emotions with more positive ones your perception of your pain will change and the amount of pain you experience will decrease.

Thinking positively is difficult and takes effort. However, if you can accept that there is no instant or total cure for your pain then you can take steps to regain control over it and your life. Some examples of more positive thoughts can be found in Table 8.2.

TENS machines

Transcutaneous electrical nerve stimulation, commonly known as TENS, is a treatment that was developed after it

Table 8.2 Positive thoughts to help overcome pain

Negative thoughts	Positive thoughts
This pain is terrible. I don't know how much longer I can cope.	I've had pain like this before and it does settle down eventually.
I can't do that job because I'm in too much pain.	I'll do it later when the pain dies down.
I can't play my favourite sport because of my pain.	I'll find other forms of exercise that don't cause so much pain.
My pain is destroying my life.	My pain is better in the morning so I'll use that time to do one new thing each day.

was observed that pain symptoms often eased when electricity was applied to the skin at the site of the pain. A TENS unit is a small battery-operated machine that is clipped onto a belt or placed in a pocket. Two small electrodes that are stuck onto the skin at the site of the pain run from the battery. The electrical impulses emitted from the battery are transmitted through the electrodes. They stimulate the nerves which in turn alleviate the pain. The intensity and rate of the impulses can be regulated by a dial located on the machine.

Acupuncture and acupressure

Acupuncture and acupressure are forms of treatment for pain involving selected points on the body (see page 100 in Chapter 7).

Shiatsu

Shiatsu is a variation of acupressure where pressure is applied to points of the body to relieve pain (see page 100 in Chapter 7).

Reflexology

Reflexology uses foot massage to treat related areas of the body (see pages 98–9 in Chapter 7).

Pain clinics

Pain clinics can help you learn to manage your chronic pain by providing you with access to expert advice, support and a personally tailored program. Although most people using pain clinics suffer from injuries following work and motor car accidents, there are clinics that provide specialised programs for women with chronic endometriosis.

Some pain clinics are run by major public and private hospitals while others are run by private specialists. All have multidisciplinary programs involving doctors, psychologists, physiotherapists, occupational therapists and nurses. The team approach is used to deal with the difficulties resulting from your chronic pain and to teach you coping strategies and how to manage your analgesics. Therapies offered include manipulation, massage, exercise, relaxation, electrostimulation, acupuncture, meditation and individual or group counselling.

9
Infertility and pregnancy

Despite the impression given by some doctors, endometriosis does not necessarily mean infertility. In fact, many women with endometriosis go on to have a baby without difficulty or have already had children when diagnosed. In addition, many infertile women with endometriosis do eventually have a successful pregnancy, although it may take time. This chapter looks at infertility, miscarriage and pregnancy in relation to endometriosis. A reading list on page 120 suggests several books that provide general information on infertility and its treatment.

Endometriosis and infertility

The issue of endometriosis and infertility has caused much controversy within the gynaecological profession over the last decade. Today, most gynaecologists agree that there is a link between endometriosis and infertility, but the nature of the link is not known. In particular, it is not known if endometriosis does cause infertility: it could be that endometriosis causes infertility, or it could be that an unknown factor causes both the endometriosis and the infertility, or it could simply be a coincidence that the two conditions are sometimes found together.

Prevalence

In the past, it was often said that 30–50 per cent of women with endometriosis were infertile. However, these figures are based on studies done in the 1930s and 1940s. Since no reliable surveys have been carried out recently, the current prevalence (or frequency) of infertility in women with endometriosis is not known. However, it is likely that endometriosis-related infertility is less common than was previously thought.

Causes

It is not known if endometriosis causes infertility. However, the exception to the rule is when the endometriosis is severe enough to cause damage to the organs of the pelvic cavity, resulting in a blockage of one or more stages of the process of conception. For example, if the ovaries are covered in adhesions that prevent the ovum escaping from the surface of the ovary, or if the fallopian tubes are blocked by adhesions that stop the passage of the sperm and ovum to the uterus. However, such damage is found in only a small proportion of women with moderate to severe endometriosis.

In almost all women with minimal or mild endometriosis and most women with moderate or severe endometriosis there is no damage to the pelvic organs. Therefore, if endometriosis causes infertility it must be the result of other factors.

Over the years, gynaecologists and scientists have tried to find out what might cause endometriosis-related infertility. In doing so they have studied many aspects of endometriosis and the female reproductive process. Among other things they have studied the processes involved in ovulation, fertilisation and implantation; the chemical composition of the fluid in the pelvic cavity; the chemicals secreted by the endometrial implants; and the immune system of the pelvic cavity. From time to time, abnormalities have been found in some women with endometriosis-related infertility and theories have been put forward to explain how the abnormality might cause infertility in those women.

However, so far, none of the theories satisfactorily explains how endometriosis causes infertility in all women with endometriosis-related infertility.

Treatment

Although it does not guarantee a pregnancy, surgery is believed by many gynaecologists to be the most effective treatment for women with endometriosis-associated infertility as it significantly improves the chances of conception. It appears to be effective for all classifications of the disease—that is, minimal, mild, moderate and severe endometriosis—and has the added advantage that it can be done at the time of diagnosis.

Surgery for endometriosis-associated infertility generally aims to remove any visible implants, nodules, endometriomas and adhesions, and repair any damage caused by the disease. The success of laparoscopy and laparotomy for minimal and mild endometriosis appears to be similar. However, for moderate and severe endometriosis pregnancy rates seem to be better after laparoscopy rather than laparotomy.

A recent large and well-designed trial of surgical treatment for women with minimal and mild endometriosis found that 31 per cent of the women who had laparoscopic surgery became pregnant within six months of their surgery. In contrast, only 17 per cent of those who did not have surgery achieved a pregnancy in the same time.

Hormonal treatment does not improve pregnancy rates in women with endometriosis-associated infertility so it is not regarded as an effective treatment. Furthermore, as pregnancy is not possible while on hormonal treatment, any attempt to become pregnant must be postponed until after treatment.

If you are unable to conceive following surgery, you may choose to try assisted reproductive technologies such as IVF (in vitro fertilisation) or GIFT (gamete intrafallopian transfer) to help you fall pregnant. However, before beginning any of these treatments it is essential that your endometriosis be properly treated. Some of the drugs used in these treatments markedly increase the level of oestrogen in the body, which may lead to a flare-up of any endometriosis present. The drugs that may cause problems include Clomid, Metrodin HP and Puregon. In addition, you are more likely to conceive if your endometriosis has been treated.

Subsequent pregnancies

Unfortunately, if you have had trouble conceiving, having a successful pregnancy does not necessarily mean that you will be able to conceive again. Some women with endometriosis-associated infertility are not able to become pregnant a second time.

Miscarriage

Before the 1990s, gynaecologists generally believed that miscarriage was more common in women with endometriosis. However, studies done in the 1980s and 1990s have shown that the rate of miscarriage in women with endometriosis is the same as for women without endometriosis.

Endometriosis and pregnancy

Pregnancy is usually assumed to lead to an improvement or remission of the symptoms of endometriosis during the pregnancy, particularly during the latter months. However, this is not always so as some women experience a worsening of symptoms, particularly during the first three months of pregnancy.

It is generally believed that the beneficial effects of pregnancy are due to the high level of progesterone produced during pregnancy. It is thought that the hormone suppresses the growth and development of the endometrial implants, causing them to gradually degenerate and waste away. The effects may also be due to the absence of menstruation during pregnancy.

The worsening of symptoms experienced by some women in the first few months of pregnancy may be a result of the high level of oestrogen produced during this stage of pregnancy. This increased level of oestrogen causes a temporary stimulation of the growth of the endometrial implants and hence a worsening of symptoms. Sometimes, the worsening of symptoms is due to stretching and pulling of adhesions as the uterus enlarges.

For many women the beneficial effects of pregnancy are only temporary. Many women—around 50–60 per cent—will experience a recurrence of their disease and its symptoms within five years and some will experience a recurrence soon after resuming their periods.

Breastfeeding

Many women with endometriosis are able to maintain the remission of their symptoms after pregnancy if they breast-feed their newborn child. Regular breastfeeding inhibits ovulation and the release of oestrogen by the ovaries, which in turn suppresses the growth and development of the endometrial implants.

Pregnancy as a cure

Many women are told by their doctors that pregnancy is a cure for endometriosis. Unfortunately, this is a myth that is still perpetuated by many GPs. The reality is that although pregnancy often leads to a temporary remission, it seldom cures endometriosis permanently. The myth appears to have arisen from the impressions and speculations of some of the early gynaecologists who had a special interest in endometriosis. In general, even those gynaecologists did not claim that pregnancy was a permanent cure. Rather, they said that pregnancy generally led to an improvement in the condition and usually delayed its recurrence.

Further reading

The following books contain detailed information on infertility, infertility investigations, infertility treatments, reproductive technologies such as IVF and GIFT, and the emotional aspects of infertility. They can be obtained from good bookstores. The exception is *Patient letters*, which is available direct from the Melbourne infertility support group, IVF Friends Inc. To buy a copy of the book, send a cheque for $18.50 to IVF Friends Inc, GPO Box 482G, Melbourne, 3001.

Brown, Loraine. 1998 *Why me?: The real-life guide to infertility*, Simon & Schuster, Sydney.
IVF Friends. 1995 *Patient letters: Personal experiences of IVF*, IVF Friends, Melbourne.
Jansen, Robert. 1997 *Getting pregnant: A compassionate resource to overcoming infertility*, Allen & Unwin, Sydney.
Powell, Susan & Stagoll, Helen. 1992 *When you can't have a child: Personal stories of living through infertility and childlessness*, Allen & Unwin/Drummond, Sydney.
Wood, Carl & Kovacs, Gabor. 1996 *Infertility: All your questions answered*, Hill of Content, Melbourne.
Wood, Carl & Riley, Robyn. 1992 *IVF: In vitro fertilisation*, Hill of Content, Melbourne.

10

Young women, teenagers and endometriosis

Today endometriosis is being diagnosed in teenagers and young women more commonly than in the past. There is also some evidence that more teenagers are developing the condition. However, very little information about endometriosis has been written with young people in mind. This chapter is especially for teenagers and young women aged 14 to 23.

Period pain and endometriosis

Many teenagers will have some discomfort with their periods, but debilitating pain is not normal and generally means that something is wrong. There are two types of period pain. Gynaecologists call them primary dysmenorrhoea and secondary dysmenorrhoea.

Primary dysmenorrhoea is the most common form of period pain in teenagers. It tends to develop after a year or two of having relatively pain-free periods and is a cramping pain that occurs for the first day or two of the period.

The pain may be accompanied by nausea, vomiting, diarrhoea, dizziness or fainting. It is caused by excessive amounts of chemicals known as prostaglandins that cause the uterus to contract too strongly during the period. Primary dysmenorrhoea can usually be alleviated by taking non-steroidal anti-inflammatory drugs such as Ponstan and Naprogesic, or by taking the oral contraceptive pill.

Secondary dysmenorrhoea is period pain that is due to an underlying disease such as endometriosis. In the case of endometriosis, the pain may start with the first period or at any stage during the teenage and young adult years.

Endometriosis is a complex disease that can have many symptoms. You may suspect endometriosis if you have one or more of the following symptoms:

- pain when you have your period
- pain when inserting a tampon
- pain when going to the toilet (especially at the time of your period)
- pain when having sex
- pain in your stomach (not necessarily at the time of your period)
- pain in your lower back.

You may especially suspect endometriosis if your symptoms are:

- so bad that you miss school, work or sport
- so painful that you have to stay in bed
- not helped by taking painkillers such as Panadol
- not helped by taking non-steroidal anti-inflammatory drugs such as Ponstan or Naprogesic
- not helped by taking the oral contraceptive pill
- occurring at the same time every month
- gradually getting worse.

If you said to yourself 'That's me' when you read the list of possible symptoms, then you should see a GP to have your symptoms investigated.

When you visit your GP, he or she will want to know how you feel throughout your menstrual cycle. Be sure to give as much information as possible. Write down the details beforehand if necessary. You will be asked how long your period pain lasts, how severe it is and whether it restricts your normal activities. You should also be asked if you have any other problems at the time of your period, such as heavy bleeding, lower back pain, or pain when you go to the toilet. If you are not asked these questions and you have any of these problems, you must tell the doctor. If you are sexually active and have found intercourse painful, you should say so as this is not normal.

Your GP may suggest that you try taking a non-steroidal anti-inflammatory drug such as Ponstan or Naprogesic, or an oral contraceptive pill for six months. If either of these drugs alleviates your pain it is more likely that you have primary dysmenorrhoea rather than endometriosis. If neither of these treatments helps your pain then your GP should refer you to a gynaecologist who specialises in treating women with endometriosis. If your GP does not refer you to a gynaecologist then you may ask to see one.

The gynaecologist will ask you numerous questions about your menstrual cycle. You may be examined and tests may be done. For more information about the questions you may be asked see pages 35–6 in Chapter 3.

Although the gynaecologist may suspect endometriosis, the only way to be sure that you have the condition is to have a procedure known as a laparoscopy. This is an operation performed under a general anaesthetic in which a telescope-like instrument is inserted into a small cut just below your navel. The gynaecologist can then inspect your pelvic organs in order to find the cause of your pain. For more information about having a laparoscopy see pages 69–79 in Chapter 6.

Unfortunately, getting a diagnosis is not always a straightforward process. Many teenagers and young women are told by family, friends and even doctors that period pain is normal and part of being a woman. Getting a diagnosis may involve convincing family and doctors that there is a problem. However, if the pattern of symptoms outlined above fits you it is important that you persist in getting your symptoms properly investigated because the problem is likely to get worse rather than better. You may need to go to several GPs before you find one who will listen to you. Ask the GP if you could have endometriosis as GPs tend to forget that endometriosis may occur in teenagers and young women. If you have trouble finding a suitable GP, your nearest women's health centre may be able to suggest one.

Living with endometriosis

Living with a chronic condition is hard for teenagers, and endometriosis is no exception. This section looks at aspects of living with endometriosis, mostly using the words of five young women.

Before diagnosis

The time before diagnosis is often difficult. When everyone else seems to be having little or no trouble with their periods, teenagers with endometriosis are faced with debilitating period pain that makes them sick enough to need time in bed and time off school or work. When they seek help from family, friends and doctors, they often receive little sympathy and are told that period pain is normal and part of being a woman. As a result, they often wonder if their pain is real or imaginary. The combination of physical symptoms and lack of understanding means that self-esteem and self-confidence are often impaired.

> *Before I was diagnosed I had reached the point where I decided I had to be imagining this pain and I began to believe the standard: 'It's all in your head'. I didn't know what was within the realms of 'normal' for a period. I had no idea that the heavy bleeding I was experiencing wasn't normal. I did, however, realise that staying in bed for a week, unable to attend school and only able to walk hunched over wasn't normal. My parents were really sympathetic and took me to doctors regularly but we always met with the same response: 'Period pain is just something you have to put up with. It's*

part of being a woman, and you've only had a few periods so they'll settle down'. I was told this so often I began to believe it.

For years I had been suffering from chronic abdominal pain. No-one could tell me what was wrong—it was just part of being a woman. My friends and family just thought that I was being a whinger and that I shouldn't complain about my pains. 'Every woman suffers from period pain' was the usual response I received from people, even doctors. I felt very alone and sometimes felt that maybe I was just imagining the pain.

Before I was diagnosed I was very depressed and lonely. I didn't understand my feelings and why I was feeling so down. I thought my pain was normal but got confused when no-one else suffered the excruciating pain I did.

Diagnosis

Once a diagnosis is made most young women experience a feeling of incredible relief knowing that something really is wrong with them. However, that feeling of relief is often followed by feelings of frustration, confusion and anger when they start to realise that endometriosis can be a long-term condition with no easy solutions.

After diagnosis I felt immense relief. I remember my gyno telling me that I had endometriosis [endo] and some adhesions which explained the heavy bleeding and pain I was experiencing. I remember thinking 'Fantastic! There really is something wrong with me and it's NOT all in my head!'

After my first laparoscopy I was a very relieved person. I wanted to shout 'I told you so' to everyone who had labelled me a hypochondriac. Although I was relieved I was also very scared. I had never heard of endo and I certainly didn't know what it was and how it had affected my body.

I was diagnosed at 14. I remember, vaguely, a doctor speaking to me in recovery, telling me that I had endometriosis. The rest of what he said was a mystery. I was scared and in a great deal of pain. When I later had the opportunity to ask some questions and voice my fears, I was told that I may never have children. The thought terrified me and I felt an immense sense of loss.

Immediately after diagnosis there was immense relief but then I was faced with decisions I was simply too young to deal with. I was only 17. The decisions I had to make were way beyond any 17-year-old. They made me grow up incredibly fast. At 17 I was no longer 'living life to the fullest'. Why did I have the burden of all this decision making that could affect the rest of my life? I was still only a kid!

My diagnosis only proved what everyone had been telling me and what had been in the very back of my mind since my sister had been diagnosed five years earlier. Now, six months after diagnosis, I still haven't considered how the disease may affect me for the rest of my life.

Symptoms

Endometriosis is more than just a collection of symptoms—it affects your whole life.

Living with my endo symptoms, such as back pain, abdominal pain, aches and pains in my legs, put a real strain on everyday life. It made getting out of bed more strenuous and difficult—especially on bad days. Being at school or work with my pain made me tired and irritable, and even just getting through the day was unbearable.

I guess the worst symptom is the tiredness. Even when the pain isn't there, I'm tired. I don't go out much and when I do I leave early. If I do have a late night I pay for it later in the week because I usually develop a migraine.

When endo 'attacks' it is the most horrible experience: extreme pain, nausea, backache, and an awful feeling of yuk! that leaves you bedridden, popping pills and hugging hot water bottles. As you experience the pain it does get easier to cope with (one thing I can't say for nausea!).

My pain put a lot of pressure on my relationship with my boyfriend. He felt there was nothing he could do to help ease my pain and felt very useless. All he could do was hold me or just be around in case I needed help getting to the toilet or if I needed a drink, etc.

Treatments

Some young women only ever need one course of treatment but others, like the women who wrote these stories, undergo a gamut of therapies and the emotional roller-coaster that can go with them.

Luckily, I haven't been on as many treatments as some teenagers. The worst hormonal treatment I've been on made me terribly nauseous and depressed so I took it for only a short time.

Constantly living on painkillers for pain relief is not only expensive but it also leaves you feeling lousy. Some days I felt like my body should rattle from all the pills I had taken.

Being on all the different hormonal drugs put a lot of stress and strain on my body. Swapping and changing drugs to find one that suited me left me feeling empty, sick, tired, depressed, moody and fed up. Some drugs felt like they changed my personality. Some made the pain feel worse. Some helped the pain but gave me other problems such as headaches. I even tried taking herbal medicines to reduce the side effects but nothing seemed to help and again I was taking more pills.

Relationships with parents

Good relationships with parents are vital for teenagers with endometriosis. They rely heavily on their parents for support and understanding when they are not feeling well and when they have to make decisions about treatment.

My relationship with my parents allowed me to survive. They were, and still are, always there for me. They are completely understanding. But, I felt so sorry for them. I could see the pain in their eyes: the feeling of utter helplessness. They had to watch their 'little girl' go through immense pain and misery, and there was nothing they could do except keep going to doctors and being there for me.

My twin sister began menstruating a year before me but she never had any trouble or pain. This, of course, led my parents, especially my father, to believe I was making up my pain to get out of things. My parents split up when I was 13, and that's when Mum really started to believe that something might be wrong. Before then my relationship with Mum was very unstable. We fought constantly and hurt each other mentally and emotionally. Once I was diagnosed with endometriosis Mum became my best friend. She has helped me make every decision along the way, and supported and encouraged me never to give up.

My relationship with my parents is very close and they are really supportive but even they have their limits. I don't think they could understand how much all the medication I was on was affecting me.

Relationships with friends

Relationships with friends often suffer before diagnosis when the teenager's friends—like most people in our community—are not very sympathetic towards her problems. However, relationships usually improve when there is a name for her problems and when the young woman herself understands her condition well enough to explain it to her friends.

My relationship with my friends became very strained. I was the only person who had endometriosis and they didn't understand what it was. I think they thought that I was a hypochondriac as I wasn't at school much and even when

I was there I was usually sick. I now have very supportive friends who take the time to listen and try their best to understand, which makes the disease easier to deal with. It's difficult when people don't understand how moody you can become and how sometimes you're just not up to going out.

Being at an all-girls school made it difficult to deal with painful periods as most of the girls didn't suffer from cramps or pain. My close friends thought I was just making a lot of it up but once I was diagnosed they soon realised I was being truthful about my pain. They couldn't understand why I couldn't go out partying all the time and why I spent at least two to three days a month in bed with a hot water bottle. It was a very hard time for me as I wanted to be accepted by my friends and didn't want to be seen as a party pooper. A lot of the time I did end up going out, even though the pain was bad or the bleeding was very heavy, just so I could be part of the group. Nowadays, I tell my friends exactly how I am feeling, and if I don't feel up to going out I tell them the truth. They know that I must be in a lot of pain to stay home because I usually try very hard to go out and do normal activities as I don't want my endo running my life.

There has been no reason why my friends at university have had to find out about my diagnosis. At the end of first year I was fine. During the holidays I was investigated, and I recuperated and returned to university the same as I left.

Coping

Living with endometriosis involves learning to cope with the physical and emotional consequences of the disease. Each young woman develops her own mechanisms.

The best way to cope with endo is to know your body well and listen to it. Pain is not a natural condition and it's your body's way of telling you that there is something wrong. Never let the pain or the emotional or mental strain beat you but don't be afraid to ask for help along the way or to try something new. Personally, I have found that a fairly general formula of eating well, exercising regularly, and getting plenty of sleep is the best way to cope.

My best coping mechanisms are talking to people and receiving their support. Talking about endo is one of the best things you can do as it allows you to express the anger, hurt and other feelings you may be experiencing. Talking to people with endometriosis is great as it makes you feel you are not alone and you can share stories and ideas on how to cope. My other coping mechanism was trying some alternative therapies. I went to yoga, which was great for relaxing my body and easing some of my stress, and I also had acupuncture, which was a great pain reliever.

One of the first things I did after I was diagnosed was to find out as much information as I could on my disease. I went to libraries, read newspapers, asked my doctor for information, and contacted the Endometriosis Association to gain support from other sufferers. I also learnt more about my body and the female anatomy. This helped me very much when I was at the doctor's surgery as I knew what he was talking about. I spoke to lots of people with the disease so I didn't feel alone. I spoke to friends and family and tried to get them to learn more about endo so they could understand what I was going through. My boyfriend came to meetings and doctors' appointments to learn more about the disease to help support me with everyday life.

Moving on

After a young woman has been diagnosed with endometriosis it usually consumes her life for a while as she learns about the condition and how to cope with it. However, it is important that she does not let it consume her life forever. At some stage she must move on—in her own way.

Endometriosis can be a vicious cycle and at the moment I'm at the beginning again. However, in the five years since my diagnosis I have learnt so much about my body, about this condition, and about how I can help myself and others. I'm no longer bitter. For a long time I asked 'Why me?' I realise now that there is no place for negativity in trying to beat this illness. For the time being I simply want to make the most of what I have at the moment and try not to think too deeply about the future. I feel I'm strong enough now to deal with anything that comes my way.

Moving on is an interesting concept that has to be looked at on many levels. You can't just 'move on'—you have to take things one step at a time. Eight years down the track I am still in the process of moving on—one step at a time.

To move on from endometriosis I have had to find other aspects in my life to concentrate on. For example, school, work, friends and social activities. Making sure endometriosis is not a focus of my life makes it easier to deal with. I allow myself to get upset but then I move on to what I need to do and what I want to achieve without my illness interfering with my life.

Accept the disease and listen to your body. Remember it is your body—trust your instincts and don't be afraid to take control. It is much easier said than done, but it IS possible.

I haven't given myself time to grieve, that is, cope with all the implications that this disease may cause, simply because the mere thought of it makes me sad.

Working positively with doctors

One of the most important things you have to do is find a GP and a gynaecologist you can trust and work with. You need doctors who you know will listen to you, who you feel comfortable talking freely with, and who can help you make decisions. If you are not getting the support you need or you are not happy with your GP or gynaecologist, find a different person. Talk to family, friends, other sufferers, or your nearest Endometriosis Association or women's health centre to see if they know someone who might be more suitable. For more information see pages 153–6 in Chapter 12.

To get the best out of your doctors you need to tell them what is happening to you. Pay attention to your body and the signals it sends you so that you can discuss them with your doctor. Remember, it is *your* body and you know when something is wrong. Keep a journal if need be so that you can remember all the details when you visit your doctor, especially if you feel uncomfortable talking on a one-to-one basis. You might like to record details of your menstrual cycle, your pain, and your feelings and emotions. For more information see pages 149–51 in Chapter 12.

When you visit your doctors, do not be embarrassed to ask lots of questions. No question is too silly or irrelevant. If you think it is important then it deserves an answer. It can be helpful to write down your questions so that you do not forget them. If you have any concerns at all about your endometriosis, raise them with your doctors.

It is important for teenagers to have input into decisions about their treatment. Your input will increase as you get older and become more independent. From time to time you may need to remind your doctors that you want more input. Regardless of how independent you want to be, listen carefully to your doctors' advice before making any important decisions.

What you can do

Living successfully with endometriosis involves effort and changes in the ways you think and act, but the effort is worthwhile. The advice in the following pages comes from five young women who have been living with endometriosis for several years.

Probably the most important thing you can do for yourself is to get accurate information about endometriosis and its treatments. Read as many books and pamphlets as you can and join your nearest endometriosis support group so that you have access to the latest information. When you understand the condition, you can appreciate how it is affecting you and how to live with it. You will also comprehend the words and ideas your doctors use, and you will be able to talk more confidently with them.

Remember that you are not alone. Seek as much support as you need. Get help with managing your pain and other symptoms, talk about your symptoms, talk about your feelings, and talk about your worries. Ask for and accept support from your parents or other adults, sisters, brothers, friends, teachers, fellow workers. Remember, they will be able to support you better if they know about endometriosis. Tell them about the condition and its impact on you. Contact the nearest endometriosis support group so you can get support from others with the disease. Try to find other young sufferers so that you can talk to young women your own age. For more information see pages 144–6 ('Coping') and pages 153–6 ('Support groups').

Accept that you have a condition that may affect you for a long time. Get to know your body and listen to the signals it sends you. Learn what each pain means and what you need to do in order to cope. Forgive yourself for doubting your pain. Be nice to yourself when you have bad days and do not push yourself when you are not feeling well. Remember, it is your body so trust your instincts. Do not be afraid to take control by doing what you think is right for you.

Do your best to find the right treatment regime for you. This may take some trial and error but it will be easier if you are well informed about the possible options. Listen to your doctors and parents and carefully consider their advice before choosing your treatment. Think of your whole lifestyle as being part of your treatment regime. Make sure that you eat well, exercise regularly, and get plenty of rest and sleep.

Try not to let the pain overpower you. Take enough painkillers to manage your pain but no more. If your pain is not being controlled by painkillers, seek help from your GP and gynaecologist. Where possible, use non-drug forms of pain relief—see pages 109–14 in Chapter 8. Experiment with the various therapies until you find one or two that work for you. If the pain is controlling your life, consult a pain clinic.

Resist making endometriosis an excuse for opting out of something you do not want to do. If you are genuinely not well do not hesitate to tell people why you cannot do it. Lastly, when you are feeling well go for it! Enjoy life!

What parents can do

Having a daughter with endometriosis can be very frustrating and heartbreaking. However, it is important that you adapt quickly to your daughter's situation so that you can provide her with the support she needs to enable her to cope and move on.

Accept the fact that your daughter has endometriosis but do not wrap her up in cottonwool. Realise that she will have good and bad days. There will also be days when she wants your help to work through her problems and days when she would prefer to deal with them herself. Help her learn to live within her limitations.

Help your daughter to get accurate and up-to-date information about endometriosis and its treatments. Learn as much as you can about the condition and its impact. Help her make contact with the nearest endometriosis support group and other young sufferers if she is interested. Talk to her about her endometriosis and its impact, and her feelings and worries. However, do not push the issue if she is not ready to discuss it.

Your daughter will need help to find a GP and a gynaecologist she can trust and work with, and you can help her establish positive relationships with them. Encourage her to talk freely with her doctors and help her prepare for her doctor visits if necessary. Ask her if she wants you to go with her when she visits the doctor. If you do go, listen carefully to what the doctor says because your daughter may not remember everything that is said.

Your daughter will want to take a greater role in making decisions about her treatment as she gets older. Make sure that she has plenty of opportunities to voice her opinions and give her the amount of guidance that is appropriate for her.

Above all, join forces with your daughter and work with her to overcome her problem.

11
Feelings and emotions

Living with chronic endometriosis involves more than just living with the physical symptoms. It also means living with the gamut of emotions that accompany the disease, and these emotions can be intense. However, understanding the emotions and realising that you are not alone in feeling them can help make them easier to cope with. This chapter looks at the feelings and emotions typically experienced by women with endometriosis, especially those with more chronic and debilitating forms of the disease, and suggests some strategies to improve your quality of life.

Before your diagnosis

Women who have been living with endometriosis for a long time before being diagnosed typically experience bewilderment, fear and frustration in the lead-up to their diagnosis.

Although the first symptom of endometriosis is usually period pain, over time a range of other symptoms gradually develops. Not understanding why you have developed symptoms such as lower back pain, bowel problems or chronic fatigue can be very bewildering. Many women also experience self-doubt about their symptoms and typically ask themselves such questions as:

- Why can't I cope with period pain when my friends have no trouble?
- Why do I spend so much time laid up in bed?
- Am I going to have to live with this period pain for the rest of my life?

- Do I have a low pain threshold?
- Is it all in my head?
- Is there anything really wrong with me?
- Why am I always so tired?
- Am I neurotic?

Many women experience pain and unpleasant symptoms before and during their periods, but what does it mean when these symptoms are chronic? Not knowing what is wrong with you is frightening enough, but if your symptoms are severe enough that your life is being disrupted it is even more frightening to think that you may never lead a 'normal' life. Sometimes sufferers can find that fear becomes the dominant emotion as some endometriosis symptoms can mimic those of life-threatening diseases such as cancer. Another dominant emotion for those who have not yet had their endometriosis diagnosed is frustration.

Frustration

Getting your endometriosis diagnosed can be a frustrating process. Too many women have their complaints of period pain and related symptoms dismissed by GPs with throw-away comments such as 'period pain is normal', 'it's part of being a woman', 'you'll grow out of it' or 'it'll get better once you have a baby'. Many women also find that GPs underestimate the severity of their pain and appear to have little understanding of the disruption it causes to their lives. Your sense of frustration may be compounded by the fact that these responses are being offered by people that you presumed would know the answers and would be able to help you.

Even if you find a sympathetic GP who will listen to your problems, the long drawn-out process of investigation can be frustrating. For example, if you have bowel symptoms and your GP sends you to a gastro-enterologist, the tests will usually be normal. That's all very well, but it still leaves you without a diagnosis. If all you are offered is the advice, 'It's probably just an irritable bowel—eat more fibre', and you've been trying that for the past six months, no wonder you feel frustrated. Although it is worth persevering in your search for a diagnosis, the process does little for your self-esteem or your faith in doctors. You are faced with a choice of just putting up with your symptoms because no-one seems able to help you, or feeling that you do nothing else except visit doctors.

Diagnosis

In view of the time it can take to get a diagnosis, it is not surprising that being diagnosed is a major turning point in the lives of many women with endometriosis. It is also a time of mixed emotions, some of which are considered below.

Relief

Most women initially feel immense relief when they are diagnosed, especially if they have been trying to get a diagnosis for some time. At last, someone has acknowledged that there really is something wrong with you and it is not all in your head. Equally important, you now have a name for your symptoms. Now you can tell others what is wrong with you and why you have been so unreliable and difficult to get along with recently.

Although much of the initial feeling of relief is because you know that there really is something wrong, some of it is because you now can see a light at the end of the tunnel. Not only do you have a name for your symptoms, you can now imagine life without them. Now you can think about possible treatments and find out which will be the best for you. There is a tremendous feeling of relief in actually being able to *do* something to help yourself.

Confusion

Unfortunately, the initial feeling of relief is sometimes followed by confusion and fear as the woman starts to realise that endometriosis is not a simple disease that can be cured with a short course of tablets. Unfortunately, too, many women are given misleading or incomplete information by their GP, which compounds these feelings. There is still a myth that endometriosis invariably causes infertility and some young women are told that they should get pregnant as soon as possible. Such advice can cause panic and turmoil in young women who have not yet found their long-term partners or established themselves in their chosen careers. Many women find it completely overwhelming to have to make such important life decisions as well as decisions about their treatment so soon after diagnosis. It is important that you find out as much as you can about your disease and its treatment, especially if you feel that you are not receiving adequate guidance or support from your doctor. Remember, as we said in Chapter 4, any decision that you take about your treatment has to be *your* decision.

Anger

Another common emotion experienced by women after the initial feeling of relief has subsided is anger. Of course you are angry that this disease has happened to you. Of course you are angry that your complaints were ignored for so long. It is important to remember that anger is a normal part of the grieving process and you may find that some of the complementary therapies discussed in Chapter 7 help you to work through your feelings of anger.

After your diagnosis

The time following your diagnosis can be a time to restore yourself, both emotionally and physically. If you are now symptom-free, or relatively symptom-free, it can be a time of emotional healing as you rediscover the joys of life. Even if you are not symptom-free, it can still be a positive time for you, now that you know what is wrong and you are beginning to understand your illness and your options. Not surprisingly, the feelings and emotions experienced after diagnosis are affected by the severity of your endometriosis and the amount of support you receive, not just from friends and family, but from the practitioners you have approached for help. Women suffering from chronic or severe endometriosis find they experience a range of negative emotions.

Frustration and depression

A significant proportion of women have recurrences of their endometriosis. This causes frustration and depression as each time you have a recurrence, you are faced with the reality that your endometriosis has not gone away and you have to make more decisions about how to manage it and your life.

The unpredictable nature of the disease means you may not know how you are going to feel from one day to the next. This can make it very difficult for you to make firm social and work commitments and, more often than not, you will not be able to do all that you want to do. Such disruption to your everyday life and relationships is extremely frustrating.

Having to undergo treatment can also be frustrating. The treatments are not usually pleasant and almost all of them have some disrupting side effects. In addition, there is the added uncertainty of whether or not a treatment will work. An unsuccessful treatment can lead to intense disappointment and frustration. Learning to put the failures behind you and to think positively about yourself and your endometriosis is very difficult and many women experience episodes of depression.

Depression is commonly experienced by women trying to come to terms with the fact that they have a chronic illness. Depression can be caused or exacerbated by a number of factors: the stress of coping with a chronic illness that drains you of energy; the strain of living with constant pain; stressed relationships; uncertainty over your future health, wellbeing or lifestyle; the disappointment of not being able to conceive; or a combination of all these. The most important thing to remember when trying to deal with depression is that it is a phase you will get through. Depression, like anger, is a normal part of the grieving process and you must allow yourself the time and space to grieve for what your diagnosis has taken away from you. Again, some of the complementary therapies in Chapter 7 have helped women to deal with depression. The fact that you are taking control of your diagnosis and treatment means that you can overcome your depression and be a stronger person for the experience.

Isolation

Chronic endometriosis inevitably leads to some degree of isolation because you cannot participate fully in the world around you. Your sense of isolation is often made worse if your partner, family and friends do not know about endometriosis and how it affects you. Ignorance is the most common reason for people being unsupportive or unsympathetic so, although it is often difficult, you owe it to yourself to tell your loved ones about the disease and its effects on you. This knowledge will enable them to support you more effectively and protect your relationships with them.

Guilt

Many women feel guilty about the impact chronic endometriosis has on their lives and relationships. Some feel guilty because they cannot fulfil all their responsibilities to their families and their relatives have to look after them from time to time. Many women suffer terrible guilt because they cannot have a normal sexual relationship with their partner. Some feel guilty about the disruption endometriosis causes to their relationships with friends while some feel guilty because they cannot match their own or their employers' expectations at work.

Unfortunately, many women have the added guilt of the possibility that they may have passed endometriosis on to their daughters. For them, their daughters' teenage and early adult years are fraught with anxiety as they carefully watch for the first signs of endometriosis.

There is no 'quick fix' to get rid of the guilt that affects so many women, although some women find that complementary therapies are helpful (see Chapter 7). It is important that loved ones have as much knowledge about your disease as possible, so that you can talk over your feelings with them.

Acceptance

Ultimately, every woman with chronic endometriosis has to accept her disease if she is to move on and lead a fulfilling life. However, for some women, especially those with more debilitating forms of the disease, the road to acceptance can be long and arduous. Accepting your endometriosis does not mean you have to like it. Rather, it means that you accept the fact that you have a chronic disease which you must learn to live with, rather than fight against. It also means learning to adapt your lifestyle, dreams and goals in order to accommodate the limitations imposed by your condition, without compromising your quality of life.

Acceptance will come gradually as you work your way through the feelings and emotions described in this chapter.

Initially, you will not be able to accept your disease all of the time and you will have 'relapses' into non-acceptance. You must realise that this is normal: it is not something to feel guilty about, nor does it mean that you have failed in trying to cope with your disease. In time, you will achieve an equilibrium that is right for you. It might not be right for any other woman, so you should not let anyone tell you how you should be feeling. Once you have achieved that equilibrium you will feel better, physically and emotionally, and you will be able to make the best of what life has to offer.

12
Taking control

Your endometriosis will probably impose long-term changes on your life, especially if you have chronic disease. You will move on and successfully overcome or learn to live with your endometriosis more quickly if you are able to develop good coping skills and a productive partnership with your doctors. You may also benefit from joining a support group. This chapter examines ways of coping with endometriosis, finding doctors and getting the best out of them, making decisions, and the role support groups can play in your recovery.

Coping

Coping with your endometriosis may be easy or it may need all the strength you can muster. Regardless of how easy or hard it is, take one step at a time and give yourself plenty of time to work through the difficulties. Most likely, you will not be able to deal with everything at once. It may help to choose one or two problems you want to tackle at the moment and then work out what you need to do in order to deal with them. Remember, tackling a problem does not necessarily mean solving it—it may just mean getting it under better control so that it is less disruptive to your life.

If you have recently been diagnosed it probably makes sense to focus on dealing with your endometriosis first, because if that is treated most of the other problems will disappear. You need to find a GP and a gynaecologist you can trust and work with (see pages 146–51). In partnership with your doctors, you can work out a treatment plan that takes account of your preferences and lifestyle. At the same time, you can help yourself by getting as much information as possible about endometriosis and its treatments (as you have already done by reading this book). Being informed enables you to start to understand the condition and its effect on you. It also allows you to start thinking about possible treatments.

If your endometriosis is not responding to surgical or hormonal treatment you might like to investigate complementary therapies to augment or replace your existing treatment (see Chapter 7). If pain is a major problem it may be worthwhile experimenting with non-drug forms of pain management such as heat packs and TENS machines—see pages 109–14 in Chapter 8.

If your life is being disrupted by your endometriosis, try to learn new ways of doing things and to seek help from others. It is imperative that you learn to accept your limitations and to work within them. Pushing yourself beyond your limits imposes more stress on your body at a time when it cannot cope with it. This makes it more difficult for your body to heal itself and leaves you less able to cope emotionally. Learn to pace yourself and cut down your activities to a manageable level. Learn to say 'No' when people ask you to do things beyond your capacity, and learn to delegate jobs and household chores. Let others know when you need help.

You can help your body cope better with your endometriosis by looking after your general health. Make sure you eat well, get regular gentle exercise, and plenty of rest and sleep. Make your rest time a chance to spoil yourself with a book, some pleasant music, a bath or a peaceful nap. Being as healthy and rested as possible will make it easier to cope emotionally and make you less cranky and difficult to live with.

Dealing with the feelings and emotions that accompany chronic and debilitating endometriosis takes time and lots of support. Talk about your feelings with your partner, family and friends so they know how you feel and so they can give you the most appropriate support and guidance. In addition, be prepared to ask them for support when you need it. If you want to talk to other women with endometriosis you might like to contact an endometriosis support group (see pages 153–6). To maintain your emotional wellbeing, find an enjoyable but gentle activity that allows you to escape your endometriosis for a while: be it going to a film, having a massage or going for a drive in the country. If your negative feelings have been overwhelming and seriously disrupting your life, you may need to think about seeing a counsellor.

Choosing your doctors

Managing your endometriosis is much easier if you have a GP and a gynaecologist you can trust and work with. Ideally, you will work with each of them in a partnership that respects your experience and knowledge of your endometriosis and your body as well as their medical experience and expertise.

Finding the right GP and gynaecologist can take time and effort, but it will be made easier if you do some thinking and homework beforehand. Think about the characteristics you want in your GP and gynaecologist, remembering that you may want different things for each of them. Typical questions to ask yourself are:

• Do I want a male or female doctor?
• Do I want someone young or old?
• Do I want someone who is interested only in conventional western medicine or do I want someone who is

happy to combine western medicine with complementary therapies?

- Do I want someone who has a special interest in endometriosis?
- Do I want to go to a specialist endometriosis clinic if there is one in my area?
- How far am I prepared to travel to see my doctor?

When you have considered what sort of doctors you would like, talk to family and friends, especially any who have had endometriosis, about doctors they know who may be suitable. If you are looking for a gynaecologist who is knowledgeable about endometriosis, you may like to ask your GP or women's health centre if they know of a suitable person. Listen carefully to the advice you are given and if necessary go back and ask more questions. Gather as much information as you need before making a choice.

When you have chosen a doctor you need to arrange a consultation. It can sometimes be helpful to make the appointment for a time when you are well so that the doctor can see you when you are feeling more confident and in control. However, this is not always possible. At your first one or two visits you may like to think about the following questions:

- Do they treat me with respect?
- Do they take me and my comments seriously?
- Do they give me enough time so I don't feel rushed?
- Do they appear to be interested in me and show compassion for my wellbeing?
- Do they appear to understand the impact the disease has on my life, physically and emotionally?
- Do they encourage questions and answer them fully?
- Do they explain all my options in language I can understand?
- Do I feel comfortable with them?
- Do I feel I can be honest with them?
- Do I feel I can trust and work with them?

It may take several visits before you really know if the relationship is going to work. If you know it is not going to work, go back to the drawing board and start again. You may need to try two or three doctors before you find the one that is right for you. Remember, you should feel totally comfortable with your doctors.

Realistic expectations of your doctors

If you are to work in a true partnership with your doctors you should feel able to talk freely and openly about your condition and its progress, and your feelings and concerns. You should also feel confident your doctors are listening to what you are saying.

It is essential that your doctors thoroughly explain any information about your condition, progress and treatments. You should also be given ample opportunity to discuss the information and ask questions. When recommending treatment options, your doctors should explain the reasons for their recommendations. This may take time but without such information you cannot make well-informed decisions about your management and you cannot form true partnerships with your doctors.

It is reasonable to expect that you will make the final decision about your endometriosis and its treatment and that your doctors will respect your decision even if they disagree with it. However, if you decide not to accept your doctors' ecommended option make sure that you have thoroughly evaluated it. In particular, make sure that you understand why they have recommended it and why you have decided to try something else.

There should be enough time during a consultation to ask any questions you may have. However, remember each appointment is scheduled to last a certain length of time. If you think you will need a long appointment ask for a double appointment. It may cost more but it will allow you the time to deal with all your concerns and the doctor will not be distracted thinking about the patients in the waiting room.

You should expect your doctors to talk to you in plain English. However, remember they are used to talking in medical language and they sometimes forget you do not know all the terminology. If your doctors lapse into medical language, ask them for a clearer explanation immediately.

Try to have realistic expectations of your doctors. Do not expect them to have all the answers, and realise that treating stubborn endometriosis can be frustrating for them as well as for you.

You can expect your gynaecologist and your GP to have quite different roles in your care. Your gynaecologist will focus almost exclusively on your endometriosis and your general gynaecological health. In contrast, your GP will have a more holistic approach and will be more interested in your overall health and wellbeing. Your GP will probably be less informed about endometriosis. However, your GP should be kept up to date about your progress and treatment through letters from your gynaecologist.

Getting the best out of your doctors

You will get the best value from your doctors if you can work with them in a partnership. You and your doctors need to combine your respective knowledge and experience about endometriosis and your body so that together you can work out what is best for you.

Being well informed about endometriosis and its treatments, and having a basic understanding of the relevant medical terms will give you a head start in working with your doctors. It will enable you to understand what they are talking about and to talk to them on a more equal footing.

Giving your doctors honest and accurate information will help them immensely. Try to give them as complete a picture as possible of your symptoms, your feelings and your responses to treatment so they can get a clear understanding of your condition and progress. Report any new symptoms no matter how trivial they seem.

It may be helpful to keep a diary of your endometriosis history so you can remember everything you need to tell your doctors. The diary could include a record of new symptoms, pain, bleeding and days off sick as well as a summary of your long-standing symptoms, laparoscopies and treatments.

When discussing your treatment options, tell your doctors about your main goal or priority—be it controlling pain, getting pregnant or simply feeling better—so you can all work towards the same goal. Similarly, if you are not happy with any aspect of your treatment let your doctors know as they may be able to suggest modifications.

Do not forget to tell your doctors about the positive as well as the negative aspects of your progress. Like everybody else, doctors like to get positive feedback and to feel they are needed and doing something useful.

Ask as many questions as you need in order to understand exactly what your doctors are saying and recommending. Do not be afraid to ask seemingly stupid or trivial questions or to query any medical words or terms you do not understand. Such questions are essential feedback for your doctors. Your questions tell them they are not getting the message across and allow them to modify it accordingly.

If you think of any questions between appointments, write them down and take the list with you to the next consultation. You may feel you are wasting your doctor's time but, in reality, you are saving time by telling the doctor what concerns you and what you do and do not understand. This makes it much easier for the doctor to tailor the consultation to your needs.

If you are given new information during a consultation it can often help to repeat the information back to your doctor to check that you have understood it correctly. If you find it difficult to remember what has been said during a consultation, take notes. If it seems appropriate, you might like to ask your doctor if there are any photographs or diagrams he or she could show you that would illustrate what is being said. If you are being given important instructions that you may forget, ask the doctor to write them down.

Sometimes it helps to a take a partner, relative or friend with you to your consultations. They can not only be comforting moral support but they can ask questions you might not feel able to ask, and they may ask questions you had not thought of. They may also say things about your symptoms that you have not noticed and they can take notes for you. Being slightly less involved they are more likely to hear and remember what is being said and they can relay that information to you afterwards.

Making decisions

Managing your endometriosis involves making decisions about treatment. It is rare for there to be any simple, black-and-white answers about treatment. As a result, deciding which treatment to use can be difficult. Spend time and effort making the right decision—after all, it is your body and you must live with the decision.

The first stage in making a decision about your treatment is to get as much information as you can about your possible options. A good starting point is the options suggested by your doctor. Read the relevant sections of this book. Ring a helpline run by one of the larger endometriosis support groups (see pages 153–6 for support groups), or talk to women you know who have used the treatments so that you can learn about their experiences. If you are not entirely happy with the options suggested by your doctor read the treatment chapters of this book to see if there are any other options you would like to consider.

Get help and support from as many people as you need, including your GP, partner, family, friends and acquaintances with endometriosis. Use them as a sounding board to test your ideas regarding the pros and cons of each option and your general feelings about treatment. Seek their thoughts as they may have ideas you have not thought of. If necessary, go over the issues with them again.

When you are ready, go back to your gynaecologist to discuss your thoughts. If necessary, ask your doctor to explain again what he or she recommends and why, especially if you are contemplating rejecting your doctor's recommendation. Tell the doctor which treatment you want to try and why you think it will be best for you. Discussing these issues will help your doctor to understand how you feel about your treatment and allow him or her to work out what further information you may need. It will also allow you to be sure that you are taking account of all the relevant issues.

If the decision is an important or difficult one, you may want to seek a second opinion from another gynaecologist. When you seek a second opinion it is important that you get a genuine second opinion by seeking someone who is going to give you independent advice or someone who has different interests or expertise. For example, if you are trying to decide between hormonal and surgical treatment it would make sense to find someone who specialises in treating endometriosis surgically if your normal gynaecologist generally treats women with hormonal drugs.

When gathering all the information about your treatment options you may become overwhelmed and confused with so much new information, especially when you try to weigh up the options and decide which treatment is the best for you. Be kind to yourself. In most cases, delaying treatment by a few days or weeks will not make any difference to your endometriosis in the long term. Take as much time as you need to make the decision that is right for you and do not let anyone push you into a decision you do not want to make. Remember, it is your body and you are the one who has to live with the decision.

Support groups

Living with chronic endometriosis is not easy. Although you may have the most supportive partner, family and friends there will still be some things they cannot understand simply because they have not had the disease. There will probably be times when you just want to talk to another woman who has had endometriosis.

Endometriosis support groups are groups set up by women with endometriosis to provide support and information for others in similar situations. There are many groups around Australia, ranging in size from a few to over 600 members.

The main role of most groups is to provide support by organising meetings and social events where women can come together and share their experiences of living with endometriosis. It can be a very comforting and empowering experience to go to a support group meeting and talk with other women who know what it is really like to have period pain, who have spent years trying to get a diagnosis and who have tried most, if not all, of the various treatments. Most women leave a support group meeting feeling much less alone.

A few of the larger groups provide support through telephone helplines. Members of the group staff the helpline so women can ring in and talk about their experiences with someone who has endometriosis. The helplines provide an important source of support for women who are not able to attend group meetings.

The larger support groups are also valuable sources of information. They publish leaflets on a variety of topics related to endometriosis. They also produce newsletters that contain recent information about endometriosis and its treatments.

Involvement in a support group can be an important part of coming to terms with endometriosis, especially if your disease is debilitating. It is a place where you can talk about your endometriosis and its treatments, and express your hopes and fears without feeling that you are perpetually whingeing or burdening your family and friends with the same old complaints. Instead, you can share your difficulties and ways of coping with women who have been in similar situations. Being able to express your problems and concerns, and listening to the experiences of others helps you to find ways of coping, sort out your feelings, and rebuild your self-esteem—all of which are essential if you are to accept your disease and move on.

The information provided informally by support groups can also be an immense help when making major decisions. While leaflets and books such as this one can provide factual information on the symptoms and treatments, they cannot provide information on such things as how do you decide when to have another laparoscopy or what is it really like to be on Zoladex? These are the types of questions you will be faced with when making decisions about your treatment. Although support groups cannot give you any simple answers, they can allow you to talk with other women who have dealt with the same questions. Listening to these women often makes it easier to sort out your own feelings and priorities, and to make a decision that is right for you.

Most support groups also welcome partners, families and friends. This can be an important way for them to learn about the disease, particularly the emotional and social aspects. Attending the meetings enables partners and relatives to better understand the effect endometriosis has on their loved one, and can be a great opportunity for family and friends to get support, especially if a partners or family night has been organised.

Endometriosis Association (Victoria) Inc

The Endometriosis Association (Victoria) ('the Association') is the largest and oldest endometriosis support group in Australia. It was established in 1984 and has over 600 members. The Association has an active group of women who work together to provide support for sufferers and their families, and accurate and up-to-date information on endometriosis and its treatments.

The group runs a helpline for women with endometriosis. Calls are welcome from women and interested people seeking support and information. Details about support groups throughout the country can be provided. The Association also runs a support group for teenagers and younger women with endometriosis, which can be contacted through the helpline.

The newsletter, which is published four times a year, is the main vehicle for support and information to members. It contains news about the group, articles on endometriosis and its treatments, and members' personal stories. Members also have access to an extensive library of books, audio tapes and video tapes.

The Association and its helpline can be contacted by telephoning (03) 9870 0536 or by writing to the Endometriosis Association (Victoria) Inc, 37 Andrew Crescent, South Croydon, Victoria 3136.

Endometriosis Clinic

In 1991 the Association established a specialist clinic for women with endometriosis in conjunction with several Melbourne gynaecologists. The clinic offers women access to gynaecologists who have extensive knowledge and experience in diagnosing and treating endometriosis. The gynaecologists have a thorough understanding of the diversity of symptoms and problems experienced by women with the condition.

The clinic offers women a second consultation with a member of the Association who has had personal experience of endometriosis. The purpose of this consultation is to discuss your possible treatment options and to provide you with any information you may need to make well-informed decisions about the management of your endometriosis. The member of the Association will use her wide-ranging experience to talk about the potential impact of the disease and its various treatments on your life, and how you might cope with your symptoms and treatments. For further information about the clinic ring the Endometriosis Association (Victoria) Inc on (03) 9870 0536.

13

For partners, families and friends

Successfully coping and coming to terms with chronic endometriosis requires considerable support from partners, families and friends. This chapter gives insights into some of the ways you may be able to help your loved one through her endometriosis. The chapter is mainly directed at partners but most of the information is also relevant to anyone—be they a parent, sister or best friend—who wants to help. The first section deals with the universal aspects of supporting someone with chronic endometriosis, and subsequent sections deal with those aspects that are specific to partners, families and friends. The final section is aimed at sufferers to remind them of the need to respect and support their helpers.

Supporting your loved one

Being supportive to your loved one involves accepting her disease, acknowledging her pain and loss, learning about her disease, supporting and encouraging her, and accompanying her on her visits to the gynaecologist if appropriate. Some of this can be very difficult as no-one likes to have to accept the fact that a loved one is ill, especially if they are young. However, you must make some changes in the ways you think and act if you are to be truly supportive.

Accept her condition

To truly support someone with endometriosis you must first accept that she has a potentially chronic disease that will have affected her life to some degree already and may affect it further in the future. An illness such as chronic endometriosis inevitably causes emotional pain and loss along with the more obvious physical effects. There is no way you can ever completely understand the full extent of your loved one's suffering. However, you can get a reasonable appreciation if you listen to and believe what she has to say about her disease and its impact.

If you can accept the fact your loved one has a disease and you can believe what she says about her disease you will be able to support and encourage her when she needs it. However, if you cannot, she will sense your disbelief and she will probably withdraw emotionally from you because she does not feel comfortable sharing information and feelings with you. Alternatively, she may feel she has to fight to convince you how much she is suffering.

Unfortunately, many people close to a newly diagnosed chronically ill person deny their loved one's illness because they find it too painful to acknowledge that they are ill or to see them suffering. They show their denial by trying to minimise the severity of the condition, and by not wanting to hear information about the disease. Denying your loved one's illness prevents you from moving on to acceptance and giving her support and encouragement when she most needs it. It also leaves her alone and isolated when she least needs it.

Accepting your loved one's disease does not mean that you welcome it. Rather, it shows her that you care, that you have compassion for her situation, that you respect and believe in her, and, above all, that you are prepared to help her in her struggle to deal with her disease—all of which she desperately needs.

Acknowledge her pain and loss

Accepting your loved one's endometriosis also means acknowledging the pain and loss caused by her endometriosis.

You need to believe what she says about her pain. She can be honest about her pain and other symptoms if she knows she will be believed. If she can be honest about her disease she can begin to cope with it. Acknowledge the losses her chronic endometriosis has caused. For example, some of her close relationships may have been strained, she may have lost many of her friends, she may have had to abandon her study or career aspirations, or she may have had to give up her favourite sport. These losses are very real and cause deep emotional pain and mourning.

Learn about her disease

Having a good understanding of endometriosis helps you to understand what is happening to your loved one and enables you to support her more effectively. Read the earlier chapters of this book or read the leaflets produced by your local support group. Discuss what you read with her. Question her and encourage her to talk about her disease, her symptoms and her treatments so you can get a better understanding of what she is experiencing and how she feels. If she is making decisions about treatment, re-read the literature and encourage her to talk about the pros and cons of the options she is considering. Be a sounding board so that she can test her ideas and thoughts about possible treatments.

It is important to understand that treating endometriosis can be difficult and may require more than one course of drugs or surgery. Some cases of endometriosis are remarkably resistant to treatment and some women have ongoing endometriosis and repeated unsuccessful treatments through no fault of their own.

It is also important to realise that women with endometriosis often experience marked mood swings. Sometimes the mood swings are due to their hormonal treatment, sometimes they are the result of being chronically ill and tired, and sometimes they are due to unknown factors associated with their endometriosis.

Support and encourage her

For most women the two best forms of support are showing her that you care and being there for her when she needs it. This might involve holding her hand or wiping her brow when she is in pain, or listening when she needs to talk about her frustrations. Always try to show your loved one that she is not alone in her struggle. Let her know that you are happy to be involved every step of the way if she wishes.

Be willing to listen and spend time talking with her about her problems and her decisions, even if you have heard it all before. Giving her the opportunity to talk about her problems will help her resolve them more quickly and allow her to move on sooner. If you are unsure how she feels about something, ask her, and listen carefully to her response so that she feels she can give you an honest answer.

Help her explore her treatment options, be they conventional medicine, complementary therapies, or pain management techniques. When exploring options or making decisions, help her to maintain a positive but realistic outlook about her prospects for success.

Think of ways you can be supportive. For example, you might like to offer to provide some occasional or regular help with housework, gardening, heavy chores or child minding.

Accompany her

If your loved one is agreeable go with her to her consultations with her gynaecologist, particularly ones where important test results or decisions are likely to be discussed.

You can provide moral support and ask questions she might not think of or feel able to ask. You can also be a more reliable ear because you will often remember explanations and recommendations that your loved one is too over-whelmed to hear. You can then discuss the information with her when you return home.

You can also accompany your loved one if she goes to an endometriosis support group meeting. You will not only provide her with moral support but you will have the opportunity to hear other women talking about their experiences and you may have the opportunity to talk to other carers and get support from people in the same situation as yourself.

Especially for partners

Endometriosis can be particularly hard on partners, who may bear the brunt of their loved one's frustrations as well as having to care for her and take on extra responsibilities around the home. Relationships are put under great strain and partners often find themselves having to take on primary responsibility for nurturing the relationship. As a result, partners may have to draw on all their reserves of patience and goodwill.

Being the partner of someone with chronic endometriosis is demanding but try to do your best to be a supportive, understanding and thoughtful partner. Above all, believe in her and regularly reassure her that you love her, especially when she is feeling down or unwell. At the same time, do not forget that your needs and feelings are important too. In particular, do not bottle up your feelings and take time out if you need to.

Try to actively build and strengthen your relationship by honestly sharing your feelings and talking over your frustrations, concerns, aspirations and day-to-day happenings. Make finding the time to talk a high priority. Being open and honest with each other will help you to overcome the stresses imposed by the endometriosis and will help to ensure neither partner feels that their needs are being neglected.

Being the partner of a woman with chronic endometriosis can be difficult. Do not be afraid to accept or ask for help from family and friends or to seek paid help if you need it. You may need assistance with housework, cooking or childcare. If you need emotional support, you may benefit from talking to another man in your situation or seeing a professional counsellor. Try to make sure that you get the help you need, when you need it. If you allow yourself to get completely overwhelmed and out of control you will not be able to support your partner and you will place the relationship at risk. After all, prevention is usually easier than trying to pick up the pieces afterwards.

Painful intercourse

Pain during or after sexual intercourse is a common symptom of endometriosis. Unfortunately, all too often it causes the couple immense emotional pain and turmoil in addition to the physical pain experienced by the woman. Some of this can be avoided with an understanding of the problem, better communication and a little experimentation.

Painful intercourse is usually the result of stretching and pulling of endometrial implants and nodules located behind the vagina and lower end of the uterus. Sometimes it is caused by vaginal dryness as a result of hormonal treatment or following a hysterectomy in which the ovaries have been removed. The pain has been described as sharp, stabbing, jabbing or a deep ache, and it may range in intensity from mild to excruciating. Women may experience pain during intercourse, or for up to 24–48 hours after intercourse, or both. Some women experience pain with any form of intercourse but others experience it only with deep penetration. The pain may be felt only at certain times of the month, such as around the time of the period, or it may be felt throughout the month.

Dealing with painful intercourse can be a difficult and emotional task. It needs open and honest communication between the couple. It also needs both partners to be patient and understanding towards each other. In particular, both partners need to develop an awareness of the other's predicament and feelings. Without these efforts, dealing with the problem can quickly degenerate into an emotional battlefield.

The woman needs to explain the nature of her pain and how it affects her, physically and emotionally. She also needs to talk about such things as her need to love and be loved, her fear of intercourse, her fear of intimacy that may lead to intercourse, her guilt about not being able to have intercourse, her guilt about letting him down, her fear of losing the relationship to someone else, and her fear that her unwillingness to have intercourse will be interpreted as a sign of rejecting him. The man needs to talk about such things as his need to love and be loved, his frustrations at not being able to have intercourse with her, his fear of hurting her, his frustration at her emotional withdrawal during times of intimacy, and his fear that he is being rejected. Once you have discussed and resolved some of these issues you will have the foundations for moving on and finding ways of resolving the problem.

With a little experimenting, you may be able to find ways or times when you can have intercourse. If appropriate, try experimenting with different positions as some women are able to enjoy intercourse if it is shallow or if slow and gentle penetration is used. You may like to try experimenting with foreplay and artificial lubricants. Some women are able to have pleasurable intercourse if there is plenty of foreplay to stimulate the natural lubricants in the vagina or if a lubricant such as KY Jelly is used.

Similarly, it may be appropriate to try experimenting with the timing of intercourse. Some women find that intercourse is pleasurable at certain times of the month, such as in the week after ovulating or in the two weeks after having a period. If you can identify the times when intercourse is pain-free, make that time of the month a special time to enjoy intimacy together.

If you experience pain during intercourse it is important that you tell your partner immediately so that he can stop. Trying to conceal the pain will usually result in you unconsciously withdrawing from him, which may be perceived as rejection. In the long term it may lead to hesitancy on your part regarding any intercourse, which will place unnecessary stress on the relationship. It is better to be open and honest at the time so that you and your partner can learn which situations create pain. That way you can learn which situations to avoid so that you can both have pleasurable and satisfying intimacy together.

Even with the most patient and sensitive experimentation, some women will not be able to experience pain-free intercourse because of their endometriosis. If this is the case you need to experiment to find other ways of sharing intimacy and lovemaking—remember, intercourse is not the only way of being intimate. Lying in bed together, kissing, hugging, holding, stroking, massaging and mutual masturbation can be just as pleasurable as intercourse if you want it to be.

Especially for families

Having relatives who can help out and be supportive is often critical for women with chronic endometriosis, who are under great stress trying to cope with their illness and keep up with all their responsibilities, especially if they have children. In addition, they often lose some of their friendships and the support networks that accompany them.

As a result, women with chronic endometriosis may become more dependent on family members for support.

If you are able to provide practical or emotional support you can be a wonderful asset for your relative. You might like to offer to help out from time to time with a few chores. However, realise that initially she may feel uncomfortable having to be more dependent on you. Read about endometriosis and its treatments and talk to her about what you have read. She can then talk to you about her endometriosis and concerns if she wishes. If she is hesitant to talk respect her privacy but let her know that you are willing to listen when she is ready to talk.

Especially for friends

Friendships develop and flourish when people spend time with each other, do enjoyable things together, and attend to each other's needs. Having chronic endometriosis inevitably leads to a loss of friends because the sufferer is unable to spend as much time and energy maintaining her friendships. The problem is often worse for younger women. Most of their friends have never experienced long-term illness so they do not understand the difficulties that go with it and they do not make as much effort to maintain the friendship. Consequently, younger women with debilitating endometriosis may lose contact with many of their friends and become isolated.

If your friend is unwell, one of the most worthwhile things you can do for her is just to be there as a friend. Making the effort to maintain the friendship through regular telephone calls and the occasional visit will make a big difference to her life. She will value talking to someone her own age and keeping in touch with what you and her other friends are doing. If you can, helping her to maintain contact with her old friends will also be extremely valuable.

Even an occasional hour or two with friends is important when you are ill and isolated.

Especially for sufferers

Having caring and reliable support people is essential for any woman with chronic endometriosis. However, it is easy to forget that those helping you also need support when you are ill and trying to cope with your illness.

Your support people are one of your most important assets, so make a real effort to preserve and strengthen your relationships with them. Show them that you love them and tell them that you greatly appreciate their love, support and care. Give them positive feedback, thank them for making your life easier, and occasionally try to do something small but special for them in return.

Do not expect other people to read your mind and do not assume that you know how your support people are feeling. Be as open and honest with them as you can. Tell them how you are feeling and give them the opportunity to tell you how they are feeling.

There may be times when you are in the depths of despair. Try not to get so preoccupied with your disease that you think you are the only person in the world with problems. Remember, your partner and other support people may be having difficulties too.

When you are feeling frustrated with the ramifications of your endometriosis it can be very easy to take your frustrations out on those around you. Although there will be times when this happens, do your best not to let it happen—after all, your loved ones are already bearing many of the consequences of your endometriosis.

Tell your partner when you feel good or better and try to share some pleasurable time together, either by being intimate or just doing something enjoyable together. Similarly, on your better days, try to spend time relaxing with any family and friends who have been supporting you.

Do not forget to let your support people, especially your partner, have time out from you and your endometriosis. You need them to maintain a healthy perspective on life and to do this they need to escape your endometriosis and all its implications from time to time. Let them go out for a game of golf or a day of fishing with the boys. They will come back refreshed and better able to help you.

Glossary

abdominal cavity: The body cavity that lies between the underside of the diaphragm and ribcage and the inner surface of the pelvis. It contains the reproductive organs, the digestive organs and the urinary organs.

acute pain: Severe pain over a short period of time.

adenomyosis: A condition in which the lining of the uterus—that is, the endometrium—'grows' into the muscular wall of the uterus.

adhesions: Bands of scar tissue that bind organs or parts of organs together.

aetiology: The causes or origin of disease.

anabolic: A body-building hormone.

analgesic: A pain-relieving drug.

androgens: The male sex hormones that are responsible for producing the male characteristics such as facial hair and a deep voice.

anteverted: Tilted forward.

antibodies: Substances formed in the body which destroy foreign materials.

asymptomatic: The absence of symptoms.

atrophy: The wasting away or decreasing in size of tissue or an organ.

atypical implant: An implant of endometrium that as yet has little or no old blood deposited in it and is usually clear, white, yellow, orange or red in colour. See also **classical implant**.

Azol: A trade name of danazol. See **danazol**.

benign: Non-cancerous.

biopsy: The removal and examination of a sample of tissue to make a diagnosis.

bladder: The sac that collects and holds urine.

bowel: Part of the digestive tract from the stomach to the anus.

breakthrough bleeding: A form of bleeding from the uterus between periods which is associated with taking birth control pills and progesterone-like drugs such as Provera and Duphaston.

candidiasis: An infection caused by a fungus known as *Candida albicans.*

carbon dioxide laser: A type of laser used in laparoscopic surgery.

cauterisation: The cutting or destruction of tissue with heat using a hot instrument, an electric current, or a caustic substance. Also known as **diathermy**.

cervix: The lowest part of the uterus which extends down into and opens into the vagina.

chocolate cyst: An endometrial cyst filled with old blood and endometrium which is found on or in the ovary.

chronic pain: Pain of long duration showing little change.

classical implant: An implant of endometrium that is brown to black in colour due to the presence of old blood. See also **atypical implant**.

Clomid: An oestrogen-like drug used to induce ovulation. Also known as clomiphene citrate.

colonoscopy: Observation of the large bowel through a telescope-like instrument.

conservative surgery: Gynaecological surgery that preserves the ability to get pregnant.

corpus luteum: The yellow sac left on the ovary after the ovum has been released from the follicle. It produces progesterone during the second half of the menstrual cycle.

cyst: A closed cavity or sac, possibly containing a liquid or semi-solid substance.

D&C: The abbreviation for dilation and curettage. A procedure in which the cervix is dilated and the lining of the uterus is scraped with a spoon-like instrument known as a curette.

danazol: A drug commonly used in the treatment of endometriosis. Also known as Danocrine.

Danocrine: The tradename of danazol. See **danazol**.

definitely diagnosed endometriosis: A diagnosis of endometriosis which is made when endometriosis has been viewed or 'visualised' during a laparoscopy or laparotomy.

dense adhesions: Adhesions that are thick and unyielding.

Depo-Provera: An injectable form of the progesterone-like drug Provera, which is sometimes used in the treatment of endometriosis.

Depo-Ralovera: See **Depo-Provera**.

diathermy: See **cauterisation**.

dilation and curettage: See **D&C**.

Dimetriose: A drug used in the treatment of endometriosis.

dioxins: Pollutants that are by-products of many industrial processes.

Duphaston: A progesterone-like drug used in the treatment of endometriosis. Also known as dydrogesterone.

dydrogesterone: The chemical name of Duphaston. See **Duphaston**.

dysmenorrhea: Painful menstruation.

dyspareunia: Painful intercourse.

ectopic: Something which is misplaced or found in an abnormal area.

electro cautery: Method of destroying endometriosis by burning it.

endometrial: Refers to something that is composed of endometrium, or something that is composed of the tissue which makes up implants and cysts of endometriosis.

endometrioma: An endometrial cyst containing old blood and endometrium. May also be known as a **chocolate cyst** if it is found on the ovary.

endometrium: The inner lining of the uterus. It is also a major component of endometrial implants.

excise: To remove completely.

fallopian tubes: The two tubes that open out from the upper part of the uterus and transport the ovum to the uterus.

fibroids: Non-cancerous tumours that are found in the uterus.

filmy adhesions: Adhesions that are thin and superficial.

fimbriae: The fringed outer ends of the fallopian tubes.

follicle stimulating hormone: A hormone produced by the pituitary gland that stimulates the growth and development of follicles in the ovary. Often abbreviated to FSH.

follicle: A sac that contains, nurtures and releases the ovum.

FSH: See **follicle stimulating hormone**.

gene: Hereditary factor present in the chromosomes of cells.

gestrinone: Chemical name of Dimetriose. See **Dimetriose**.

GIFT (gamete intrafallopian transfer): A process whereby the ovum and sperm are placed in the fallopian tube via laparoscopy.

GnRH: See **gonadotropin releasing hormone**.

gonadotropin releasing hormone: A hormone produced in the brain that directs the pituitary gland to release follicle stimulating hormone and luteinising hormone. Often abbreviated to GnRH.

gonadotropins: Hormones produced by the pituitary gland that stimulate the ovaries.

goserelin acetate: Chemical name of Zoladex. See **Zoladex**.

hormone replacement therapy: Drug therapy that supplies the body with oestrogen and/or progesterone after menopause.

hormones: Chemical substances that regulate various body processes.

hypo-oestrogenic: Low levels of oestrogen in the body.

hysterectomy: The surgical removal of the uterus.

hysteroscopy: Observation of the interior of the uterus through a telescope-like instrument known as a hysteroscope.

immune system: Defence system of the body.

implant (endometrial): An island or nodule of endometrium. See **classical implant** and **atypical implant**.

implant (hormonal): A pellet of synthetic oestrogen that is inserted under the skin in hormonal therapy.

in vitro fertilisation (IVF): A procedure in which an ovum is removed from the follicle, fertilised outside the body and placed in the uterus.

internal os: The internal opening of the cervix into the uterus.

irritable bowel syndrome: A condition characterised by involuntary spasms of the large intestine.

IVF: See **in vitro fertilisation**.

labia: Two folds of skin that surround the entrance of the vagina.

laparoscopy: An operation in which the abdominal cavity and the reproductive organs are viewed or 'visualised' by passing a telescope-like instrument known as a laparoscope through a small cut in or near the navel.

laparotomy: A major operation which involves a large cut through the abdominal wall.

laparoscope: A telescope-like instrument used to view contents of the pelvic cavity.

laser surgery: An operation involving the use of a laser beam instead of a knife to cut and destroy tissue.

laser: An extremely concentrated beam of light that can be precisely directed onto tissue to cut or destroy it.

lesion: A wound or an abnormal change in tissue or an organ of the body.

LH: See **luteinising hormone**.

ligament: A tough band of fibrous tissue that joins two areas of the body and helps to hold them in place.

luteinising hormone: A hormone produced by the pituitary gland that initiates ovulation and then stimulates the corpus luteum to produce progesterone. Often abbreviated to LH.

lymphatic system: A complex of vessels and glands that drain off and filter tissue fluid.

medroxyprogesterone acetate: The chemical name of Provera, Ralovera and Depo-Provera. See **Provera** and **Depo-Provera**.

membrane: A layer of thin elastic tissue that covers the surface of some organs and lines the cavities of the body.

menarche: The onset of menstruation.

menopause: The cessation of menstruation.

menorrhagia: An excessive flow of blood during menstruation.

menstruation: The monthly flow of blood and endometrial tissue from the uterus via the vagina—that is, the monthly period.

myometrium: Muscle layer of the uterus.

naferelin acetate: Chemical name of Synarel. See **Synarel**.

narcotics: Habit-forming drugs.

node: See **nodule**.

nodule: A small firm lump.

non-Hodgkin's lymphoma: Cancer of the lymph tissue.

non-steroidal anti-inflammatory drugs: Drugs to treat inflammation and pain.

oestrogen replacement therapy: Drug therapy that supplies the body with oestrogen after menopause.

oestrogen: A female sex hormone produced by the ovaries that stimulates the endometrium to grow and thicken.

oophorectomy: The surgical removal of an ovary or ovaries.

osteoporosis: A condition in which the bones become thin and porous, causing them to break easily.

ova: The plural of ovum. See **ovum**.

ovary: The female sex gland that produces the ovum.

ovulation: The expulsion of the mature ovum from the ovary.

ovum: The egg produced by the ovary.

palpate: The technique of examining the organs and parts of the body by probing and feeling the area with the fingers.

patent: Something that is not blocked.

PCBs: Pollutants that are by-products of industrial processes.

pelvic cavity: The part of the abdominal cavity where the reproductive organs are located.

pelvic examination: A routine gynaecological examination of the reproductive organs in which the organs and their supporting ligaments are felt or 'palpated' by the doctor.

pelvic inflammatory disease: Inflammation and/or infection of the female reproductive system—that is, the cervix, uterus, fallopian tubes and ovaries. Commonly abbreviated to PID.

peritoneal cavity: The space and organs within the abdomen and pelvis.

peritoneal fluid: The fluid that is produced in very small amounts by the peritoneum.

peritoneum: The membrane that lines the abdominal and pelvic cavities and forms a covering for the abdominal and pelvic organs.

PID: See **pelvic inflammatory disease**.

pituitary gland: The gland located at the base of the brain which secretes many hormones, including follicle stimulating hormone and luteinising hormone.

polycystic ovaries (PCO): Ovaries that contain an excessive number of follicles.

Pouch of Douglas: The area between the back of the uterus and vagina and the front of the rectum.

premature menopause: Menopause which for whatever reason occurs at an earlier age than the usual age for the menopause.

pre-sacral neurectomy: An operation in which the nerves that transmit pain from the uterus to the brain are cut. Very rarely done in Australia.

primary dysmenorrhoea: 'Cramping' type of period pain that typically affects teenagers.

progesterone: A hormone produced by the corpus luteum in the second half of the menstrual cycle which prepares the lining of the uterus for implantation of the fertilised ovum.

progestogens: Synthetic hormones that have an action like progesterone.

prostaglandin inhibitors: Drugs that suppress the action of prostaglandins.

prostaglandins: Substances produced throughout the body that control many functions in the body, including the contraction and relaxation of the muscles of the uterus.

Provera: A progesterone-like drug used in the treatment of endometriosis. Also known as medroxyprogesterone acetate.

pseudomenopause: The creation of the hormonal conditions of menopause using drugs such as danazol.

pseudopregnancy: The creation of the hormonal conditions of pregnancy using drugs such as Duphaston and Provera.

Ralovera: See **Provera**.

rectovaginal septum: The membrane that separates the vagina and the rectum.

rectum: The end portion of the large bowel.

reflux: See **retrograde menstruation**.

retrograde menstruation: The back-up or backward flow of the menstrual fluid through the fallopian tubes and out into the pelvic cavity. Also known as reflux.

retroverted: Tilted backwards.

sacrum: The large central bone at the base of the spine that forms part of the pelvis.

scavenger cells: Immune cells that destroy bacteria and other foreign material.

secondary dysmenorrhoea: Period pain due to an underlying cause such as endometriosis.

steroids: A group of hormones which includes oestrogen, progesterone and the androgens.

surgical menopause: Menopause which occurs when both ovaries are destroyed by surgery before the usual age of menopause.

Synarel: A GnRH analogue drug used in the treatment of endometriosis.

testosterone: A male hormone produced by the testes which stimulates the development of male characteristics such as facial hair and a deep voice.

tissue: Mass of cells forming one of the structures of which the body is composed.

ultrasound: A procedure in which high-frequency sound waves are used to detect abnormalities in the body.

umbilicus: Navel.

ureter: The tube that drains urine from the kidney into the bladder.

utero-sacral ligaments: Bands of tissue that help support the uterus.

utero-sacral neurectomy: An operation to cut the nerves that transmit pain from the uterus to the brain.

uterus: The hollow, muscular pear-shaped organ that carries and nurtures the foetus.

vagina: The muscular canal that connects the cervix to the external surface of the body.

vulva: The external female genital organs.

womb: Another name for the uterus. See **uterus**.

Zoladex: A GnRH analogue drug used in the treatment of endometriosis.

Index